Hope Faith & Courage

VOLUME II

Stories and Literature from the Fellowship of Cocaine Anonymous

C.A. World Service Conference-Approved Literature
Cocaine Anonymous World Service, Inc.
Los Angeles, California
2012

Twelve Steps and Twelve Traditions
reprinted with adaptation by permission
of A.A.World Services, Inc.

Cocaine Anonymous World Services, Inc.
P.O. Box 492000
Los Angeles, CA 90049-8000
www.ca.org
e-mail: cawso@ca.org

2nd Edition

Printed in the United States of America.

9 8 7 6 5 4 3

Library of Congress Cataloging-in-Publication (CIP) Data
Hope, Faith & Courage Volume II
Stories and Literature from the Fellowship of Cocaine Anonymous.

Library of Congress Catalog No. 93074413

ISBN 978-0-9791491-0-8

C.A. World Service Conference-Approved Literature

To the addict who still suffers...

PREFACE

In November of 1982, several recovering addicts met and established the first Cocaine Anonymous (C.A.) group. Since that first meeting, Cocaine Anonymous has grown significantly. In 2012, approximately 2100 groups in 25 countries around the world claimed a home in C.A. People seeking recovery have found C.A. in small towns, large cities and in cyberspace through the internet.

C.A. members are people from all walks of life and from all parts of the world. The hope is that you may find recovery as we did and stay sober, one day at a time.

At the spiritual center of Cocaine Anonymous is a message of hope, faith and courage. We wish to assure you that this is a spiritual program, not a religious one. The message of recovery does not conflict with any of our members' established religious affiliations or beliefs, or lack thereof. Our experience has demonstrated that such matters remain personal decisions for the individual member and as such, are not required for the spiritual growth that is possible as a result of working the Twelve Steps of Cocaine Anonymous.

In order for this message to be more widely available to the addict seeking recovery from addiction, this collection of stories and literature has been compiled to recount the personal experiences of C.A. members and to describe our message of recovery. These stories offer a wide variety of experiences regarding the concept of a Higher Power, a God of your own understanding. All are valid examples of our diversity and the broad, inclusive nature of the spiritual solution that solves our common problem.

Although some of the names of the drugs and methods of their use have changed over time, the need for recovery from addiction has not. To that end, it is our hope that you will find the message of recovery here in this volume of *Hope, Faith and Courage.*

No matter where you are or what fuels your addiction, **you are not alone** and **there is a solution**.

"We're Here and We're Free" ™

TABLE OF CONTENTS

Preface v
We Can Recover xi
To the Newcomer xv
Tools of Recovery xxi
... And All Other Mind-Altering Substances xxv

PERSONAL STORIES

1 **OUR HOPE, FAITH AND COURAGE** **1**
The early days of Cocaine Anonymous as experienced by two of its members.

2 **EAP TO C.A. AND HP TO LIFE** **11**
Her most life-changing moment of all was when her boss sent her to the Employee Assistance Program that began the path of living in recovery.

3 **READY FOR ANYTHING** **19**
She was looking for help to get rid of a drug problem, but what she found was an entire new way of life.

4 **SET FREE BY THE TRUTH** **27**
After being released from jail, he was still imprisoned by secrets about his addiction. Getting honest was his key to freedom.

5 **DERAILED** **33**
His life was a train wreck. Now he's living the dream.

6 **NORMAL ON THE OUTSIDE** **41**
Cocaine Anonymous taught her it was an inside job.

7 **GETTING UNSTUCK** **47**
One addict's journey from emergency rooms to the rooms of recovery.

8 **BIRTHMARK** **57**
A stray bullet was the beginning of a new life.

9 **A LIFE WORTH LIVING** **63**
By doing the best he could each day of his recovery and leaving the results up to God, he experienced a life beyond his wildest expectations.

10 **DOWNWARD SLIDE** 71
His unmanageability took him to places he thought he'd never go; recovery brought him back.

11 **CALL COCAINE ANONYMOUS, WE CAN HELP** 77
The C.A. helpline directed him to his first meeting. Through working the Steps, he has replaced a cocaine high with a spiritual connection.

12 **FINALLY HOME** 85
Blaming God for his father's death, this addict drank and drugged his way through life. Now, through C.A. and God's help, he is free from the misery, terror and pain of being a using addict.

13 **AN ATTITUDE OF GRATITUDE** 89
Practicing gratitude totally turned her attitude around, and looking for the good in her life became a reflex.

14 **INSIDE OUT AND BACK AGAIN** 101
He went from the brink of insanity to the leading edge of a beautiful adventure.

15 **A LIAR, A CHEAT, A THIEF AND A WHORE** 109
She went from the bottom of her addiction to being a proud and grateful member of Cocaine Anonymous.

16 **OUT OF DESTRUCTION AND FEAR** 115
He lied, cheated and stole his way to the bottom until his sister carried the message that led him to recovery.

17 **FROM DOMINANCE TO SURRENDER** 125
Finding a Higher Power of her own understanding allowed her to become a free and happy woman.

18 **GOD SENT A TAXI** 131
She took a ride home to Cocaine Anonymous.

19 **A RECOVERED MISFIT** 139
She discovered that her world was the right size and learned how to walk through rough times with dignity and grace.

20 **LIVING LIFE TO THE MAX** 145
Speeding through addiction, he surrendered to a new way of living, one day at a time.

21 **OUT OF THE STREETS AND INTO SOBRIETY** 151
Recovery taught this former gangster how to give up, own up, make up and grow up.

22 **LIFE LESSONS** 157
Facing challenges helped her find the strength and faith to follow her calling.

23 **AN ULTIMATUM TO GOD** 161
"Just say no" and "Just don't pick up" did not work for this addict. She finally heard the message while listening for God to answer her challenge.

24 **IN SPITE OF MYSELF** 169
It worked because she worked the Steps.

25 **MY FOREVER CLEVER MIND** 177
The simple concept of one addict helping another proved far more effective than his own best thinking.

26 **MOMENT OF CLARITY** 189
An experience of conscious contact removed his obsession to use.

LITERATURE

1 **COCAINE ANONYMOUS SELF-TEST** 197

2 **TIPS FOR STAYING CLEAN AND SOBER** 201

3 **THE FIRST 30 DAYS** 203

4 **A HIGHER POWER** 207

5 **THE HOME GROUP** 209

6 **CHOOSING YOUR SPONSOR** 213

7 **BEING OF SERVICE** 217

8 **CRACK** 221

APPENDICES

A **SUGGESTED MEETING FORMAT** 227

B **TWELVE STEPS OF COCAINE ANONYMOUS** 241

C **TWELVE TRADITIONS OF COCAINE ANONYMOUS** 243

WE CAN RECOVER

Welcome to Cocaine Anonymous. We are all here for the same reason—our inability to stop using cocaine and all other mind-altering substances. The first step towards solving any problem is admitting that there *is* a problem.

The problem, as we see it, consists of an obsession of the mind and an allergy of the body. The obsession is a continued and irresistible thought of cocaine and the next high. The allergy creates an absolute inability to stop using once we begin.

We wish to assure you that there *is* a solution and that recovery *is* possible. It begins with abstinence and continues with practicing the Twelve Steps of recovery, one day at a time. Our program, the Twelve Steps of Cocaine Anonymous, is the means by which we move from the problem of drug addiction to the solution of recovery.

1. We admitted we were powerless over cocaine and all other mind-altering substances—that our lives had become unmanageable.

2. Came to believe that a Power greater than ourselves could restore us to sanity.

3. Made a decision to turn our will and our lives over to the care of God *as we understood Him*.

4. Made a searching and fearless moral inventory of ourselves.

5. Admitted to God, to ourselves, and to another human being the exact nature of our wrongs.

6. Were entirely ready to have God remove all these defects of character.

7. Humbly asked Him to remove our shortcomings.

8. Made a list of all persons we had harmed, and became willing to make amends to them all.

9. Made direct amends to such people wherever possible, except when to do so would injure them or others.

10. Continued to take personal inventory and when we were wrong promptly admitted it.

11. Sought through prayer and meditation to improve our conscious contact with God *as we understood Him*, praying only for knowledge of His will for us and the power to carry that out.

12. Having had a spiritual awakening as the result of these Steps, we tried to carry this message to addicts, and to practice these principles in all our affairs.[1]

Cocaine Anonymous is a spiritual program, not a religious one. In C.A. we believe each individual can choose a Higher Power of his or her own. In short, a God of his or her own understanding.

No one comes into Cocaine Anonymous to find God. We came into these rooms to get rid of a terrifying drug habit. Look around this room. You are surrounded by people who came as a last resort. We came into these rooms emotionally, financially and spiritually bankrupt. We have experienced all sorts of tragedies as a result of cocaine, drugs and/or alcohol. We have lived many of the same horrors you have, yet today we are free from the misery, terror and pain of addiction.

Maybe some of us were worse off than you; maybe some of us didn't hit as low a bottom as you. Still the fact remains that those of us who are recovering have come to believe that a Higher Power of our own understanding can restore us to sanity.

There *is* a solution; we *can* recover from addiction. One day at a time, it is possible to live a life filled with hope, faith and courage.

[1]The Twelve Steps are reprinted with permission of Alcoholics Anonymous World Services, Inc. Permission to reprint and adapt the Twelve Steps does not mean that A.A. is affiliated with this program. A.A. is a program of recovery from alcoholism. Use of the Steps in connection with programs and activities which are patterned after A.A. but which address other problems does not imply otherwise. THE TWELVE STEPS OF ALCOHOLICS ANONYMOUS: 1. We admitted we were powerless over alcohol—that our lives had become unmanageable. 2. Came to believe that a Power greater than ourselves could restore us to sanity. 3. Made a decision to turn our will and our lives over to the care of God *as we understood Him*. 4. Made a searching and fearless moral inventory of ourselves. 5. Admitted to God, to ourselves, and to another human being the exact nature of our wrongs. 6. Were entirely ready to have God remove all these defects of character. 7. Humbly asked Him to remove our shortcomings. 8. Made a list of all persons we had harmed, and became willing to make amends to them all. 9. Made direct amends to such people wherever possible, except when to do so would injure them or others. 10. Continued to take personal inventory and when we were wrong promptly admitted it. 11. Sought through prayer and meditation to improve our conscious contact with God *as we understood Him*, praying only for knowledge of His will for us and the power to carry that out. 12. Having had a spiritual awakening as the result of these Steps, we tried to carry this message to alcoholics, and to practice these principles in all our affairs.

TO THE NEWCOMER

WHO IS A COCAINE ADDICT? Some of us can answer without hesitation, "I am!" Others aren't so sure. Cocaine Anonymous believes that no one can decide for another whether he or she is addicted. One thing is sure, though: every single one of us has *denied* being an addict. For months, for years, we who now freely admit that we are cocaine addicts thought that we could control cocaine when in fact it was controlling us.

"I only use on weekends," or
"It hardly ever interferes with work," or
"I can quit, it's only psychologically addicting, right?" or
"I only snort, I don't base or shoot," or
"It's this relationship that's messing me up."

Many of us are still perplexed to realize how long we went on, never getting the same high we got at the beginning, yet still insisting, and believing—so distorted was our reality—that we were getting from cocaine what actually always eluded us. We went to any lengths to get away from being just ourselves. The lines got fatter; the grams went faster; the week's stash was all used up today.

We found ourselves scraping envelopes and baggies with razor blades, scratching the last flakes from the corners of brown bottles, snorting or smoking any white speck from the floor when we ran out. We, who prided ourselves on our fine-tuned state of mind! Nothing mattered more to us than the straw, the pipe, the needle. Even if it made us feel miserable, we had to have it.

Some of us mixed cocaine with alcohol or other drugs, and found temporary relief in the change, but in the end, it only compounded our problems. We tried quitting by ourselves, finally, and managed to do so for periods of time. After a month, we imagined we were in control. We thought our system was cleaned out and we could get the old high again, using half as much. This time, we'd be careful not to go overboard. But we only found ourselves back where we were before, and worse.

We never left the house without using first. We didn't make love without using. We didn't talk on the phone without coke. We couldn't fall asleep; sometimes it seemed we couldn't even breathe without cocaine. We tried changing jobs, apartments, cities, lovers—believing that our lives were being screwed up by circumstances, places, people. Perhaps we saw a cocaine friend die of respiratory arrest, and *still* we went on using! But eventually we had to face facts. We had to admit that cocaine was a serious problem in our lives, that we *were* addicts.

WHAT BROUGHT US TO COCAINE ANONYMOUS? Some of us hit a physical bottom. It may have been anything from a nosebleed which frightened us, to sexual impotence, to loss of sensation in or temporary paralysis of a limb, to a loss of consciousness and a trip to an emergency room, to a cocaine-induced stroke that left us disabled. Maybe it was finally our gaunt reflection in the mirror.

Others of us hit an emotional or spiritual bottom. The good times were gone, the coke life was over. No matter how much we used, we never again achieved elation, only a temporary release from the depression of coming down, and often, not even that. We suffered violent mood swings. Perhaps we awoke to our predicament after threatening or actually harming a loved one, desperately demanding imagined hidden money. We were overcome by feelings of alienation from friends, loved ones, parents, children, society, from the sky, from everything wholesome. Even the dealer we thought was our friend turned into a stranger when we went to him without money. Perhaps we awoke in dread of the isolation we had created for ourselves—using alone, suffocated by our self-centered fear and our paranoia. We were spiritually and emotionally deadened. Perhaps we thought of suicide, or tried it.

Still others of us reached a different sort of bottom when our spending and lying cost us our jobs, credit, and possessions. Some of us reached the point where we couldn't even deal; we consumed everything we touched before we could sell it. We simply could no longer afford to use. Sometimes the law intervened.

Most of us were brought down by a medley of financial, physical, social, and spiritual problems.

When we found Cocaine Anonymous, we learned that cocaine addiction is a progressive disease, chronic and potentially fatal. It fit our own experience when we heard that, contrary to popular myths about cocaine, it is possibly the most addictive substance known to man. We were relieved to be told that addiction is not simply a moral problem, that it is a true disease over which the will alone is usually powerless. All the same, each of us must take responsibility for our own recovery. There is no secret, no magic. We each have to quit and stay sober; but we don't have to do it alone!

WHAT IS COCAINE ANONYMOUS? We are a Fellowship of addicts who meet together to share our experience, strength, and hope for the purpose of staying sober and helping others achieve the same freedom. Everything heard at our meetings is to be treated as confidential. There are no dues or fees of any kind. To be a member, you only have to want to quit, and show up. We also exchange phone numbers, and give and seek support from one another between meetings.

We are all on equal footing here. There are no professional therapists offering treatment, and no one "runs" the group. Everyone in these rooms is here because he or she has a desire to stop using cocaine and all other mind-altering substances. We are men and women of all ages, races, and social backgrounds, with the common bond of affliction. Our program, called the Twelve Steps of recovery, is gratefully borrowed from Alcoholics Anonymous, whose more than 50 years of experience with substance abuse teaches us that the best human help an addict can receive is from another addict. Some of us may first come to C.A. while in a treatment program or seeking individual psychotherapy. We say, "Fine, do whatever works for you." We don't pretend to have all the answers, but experience has taught us that a recovering addict will almost certainly relapse without the ongoing support of fellow addicts.

We welcome newcomers to C.A. with more genuine warmth and acceptance in our hearts than you can probably now imagine—for you are the lifeblood of our program. In great part, it is by carrying the message of recovery to others like ourselves that we keep our own sobriety. We are all helping ourselves by helping each other.

WHAT IS THE FIRST THING? To the newcomer who wonders about the first thing he or she must do to achieve sobriety, we say that you have already done the first thing: you have admitted to yourself, and now to others, that you need help by the very act of coming to a meeting or seeking information about the C.A. program.

You are also, at this very moment, doing the next thing to stay straight; you are not taking the next hit. Ours is a one-day-at-a-time program. We suggest that you not dwell on wanting to stay sober for the rest of your life, or for a year, or even a week. Once you have decided you want to quit, let tomorrow take care of itself. Just for today, you don't have to use. But sometimes it is too much for us to project even one whole day drug-free. That's okay. Just for the next ten minutes, you don't have to use. It's okay to want it, but you don't have to use it, just for ten minutes. After ten minutes, see where you are. You can repeat this simple process as often as necessary, using whatever span of time feels comfortable. *Just for today, you don't have to use!*

In the C.A. Fellowship, you are among recovering cocaine abusers who are living without drugs. Make use of us! Take phone numbers. Between meetings, you may not be able to avoid contact with drugs and druggies. Some of us had no sober friends at all when we first came in. You have sober friends now! When you begin to feel squirrelly, don't wait. Give one of us a call; and don't be surprised if one of us calls you when we need help!

It may surprise you that we discourage the use of *any* mind-altering substances, including alcohol and marijuana. It is the common experience of addicts in this and other programs that *any* drug use leads to relapse or substitute addiction. If you're addicted to another substance, you'd better take care of it. If you're not, then you don't need it, so why mess with it? We urge you to heed this sound advice drawn from the bitter experience of other addicts. Is it likely you're different?

We thought we were happiest with our cocaine, but we were not. In C.A., we learn to live a new way of life. We say that it is a spiritual but not a religious program—our spiritual values are accessible to the atheist as well as to the devout theist.

We who are grateful recovering cocaine addicts ask you to listen closely to our stories. That is the main thing—listen! We know where you're coming from, because we've been there ourselves. Yet we are now living drug-free, not only that, but living happily; many of us, happier than we have ever been before. Few of us would trade all our years of addiction for the last six months or year of living the C.A. program of sobriety.

No one says that it is easy to arrest addiction. We had to give up old ways of thinking and behaving. We had to be *willing to change*. But we are doing it, gratefully, one day at a time.

TOOLS OF RECOVERY

There comes a time when the cocaine stops working – a time when the coke, the other drugs, and all the madness become unbearable. By then, you just can't stop, so you manage to score and somehow survive. You keep on using because, although it's killing you, cocaine has become the most important thing in your life. If you somehow, some way, get a break from it, get free for a moment with a little clarity, you will know this could be your last chance. You must stop using now, and you are really scared. You want to stay away from cocaine, but you don't know how.

If you want to be clean and sober, you can be. If you want what we have, you can have it. No matter how much cocaine you have used or how low you have sunk, you can get away and stay away from cocaine, by doing what we have done. Thousands of recovering cocaine addicts are living drug-free and owning their lives again, by actively using the tools of recovery in the program of Cocaine Anonymous. Here are some of the tools that work for us.

TOTAL ABSTINENCE Those of us who have lost control of our cocaine consumption must abstain from all mind-altering substances. It's our experience that our addiction is invariably triggered by the use of alcohol and other drugs. Just don't drink or use–no matter what.

MEETINGS We attend meetings to share our experience, strength, and hope with other recovering addicts. What we failed to do alone we can do together. We also learn valuable information about our disease and how the program of Cocaine Anonymous works in our lives. We suggest that you get a meeting directory and go to 90 meetings in 90 days.

LITERATURE The books *Alcoholics Anonymous* (the "Big Book") and *Twelve Steps and Twelve Traditions* (the "Twelve and

Twelve") of Alcoholics Anonymous are two of our most valuable tools of recovery. In addition, Cocaine Anonymous publishes numerous pieces of literature to further help the recovering addict, including our books, *Hope, Faith & Courage: Stories from the Fellowship of Cocaine Anonymous*, and *Hope, Faith & Courage Volume II: Stories and Literature from the Fellowship of Cocaine Anonymous.*

SPONSOR A sponsor is another recovering addict who has more sobriety and program experience than yourself. He or she (same sex is recommended) will help you work the Steps and should be someone you feel comfortable communicating with. We recommend that you begin looking for a sponsor immediately. You can change sponsors later if the relationship doesn't work out.

THE TWELVE STEPS Meetings may keep you sober for some time, but the Twelve Steps of Cocaine Anonymous are vital for a stable and happy recovery. The Steps of Cocaine Anonymous are the means by which we move from the problem of drug addiction to the solution of recovery. We learn about the Steps by reading the literature, attending Step study meetings, and working with a knowledgeable sponsor.

HIGHER POWER We urge new members to explore whatever beliefs they may have in a Power greater than themselves. There are no religious requirements or beliefs necessary for membership in Cocaine Anonymous. Some of us had lost our spirituality before we came to C.A., and others of us never had any. As we recovered, many of us experienced new or reawakened spiritual feelings. It helps to be open-minded.

SERVICE One of the keys to successful recovery is getting involved. Begin by taking on tasks and keeping commitments at meetings–make coffee; help clean up; put away chairs. Help yourself by helping others.

TELEPHONE The telephone is our lifeline between meetings. Get phone numbers from other C.A. members. We are usually shy about calling at first, but we must find a way to do it. We suggest you call someone in the program daily.

ONE DAY AT A TIME The thought of making a pledge never to use again can be discouraging. We stay clean and sober one day at a time and if necessary, one hour or even one minute at a time.

PRAYER AND MEDITATION We use these tools to establish and improve our conscious contact with God, *as we understand Him.* We have found the Serenity Prayer to be very helpful:

God, grant me the serenity to accept the things I cannot change, courage to change the things I can, and wisdom to know the difference.

Make your recovery your number one priority. All your hopes and plans, even your very survival, depend on a drug-free you. Staying away from cocaine and all other mind-altering substances may be the greatest challenge you will ever face. The early period can be tough, but that doesn't mean you are not getting better. Beware of thoughts like, “I don't feel good,” or “This is not working.” Recovery is a process, and it takes time.

We hope that by using these tools you will find the same joy and freedom we have found. Just remember to be patient and keep coming back.

... AND ALL OTHER MIND-ALTERING SUBSTANCES

STEP ONE: *We admitted we were powerless over cocaine and all other mind-altering substances—that our lives had become unmanageable.*

TRADITION THREE: *The only requirement for C.A. membership is a desire to stop using cocaine and all other mind-altering substances.*

Many people come to Cocaine Anonymous thinking one of two things: "I rarely (or never) even used cocaine. I don't think I belong here," or "What exactly does the 'and all other mind-altering substances' part mean? I came to Cocaine Anonymous because *cocaine* had become a problem in my life."

Those of us who have been C.A. members for a while have heard questions and statements like this before; perhaps the words were even our own. Over time, virtually every single one of us has realized that our real problem is not cocaine or any specific drug, it is the disease of addiction.

Some of us never even used cocaine. Some of us used a variety of drugs, and for others it was combining cocaine with alcohol and/or other drugs that got us into trouble and made our lives miserable. Many of us rode drug roller coasters; there were drugs to come down with, drugs to go up with, and drugs to mellow out with.

During those times we attempted to regain control we found that any substitution or new combination inevitably created the same result. It was hard to stop and easy to get started. Experience after experience revealed that substitution was no cure. If our bodies were not absolutely free of drugs and alcohol, the obsession to use more of something was always lurking.

For example, imagine that you have just run out of one drug and cannot get any more. What would you use for a substitute? Alcohol for heroin, methamphetamine for cocaine, prescriptions for whatever, vice-versa–the list could go on and on and it really wouldn't matter. The point is that addicts like us soon find ourselves unable to stop using the substitute. Whatever drug we use, the problem of not being able to stop resurfaces, often bigger than before.

At some point we finally realize that we cannot control our use of *any* mind-altering substances. The problem isn't the drug of choice; the problem is the disease of addiction. With its Third Tradition and all-inclusive First Step, Cocaine Anonymous welcomes anyone with a drug or alcohol problem and offers a solution.

ALCOHOL AND MARIJUANA

Marijuana is a potent drug, and alcohol is a mind-altering chemical in liquid form. Many people don't realize that these are no different from any other drugs regarding the potential to get us into trouble. One drink is never enough; just as one puff, hit, fix, bump, pill or snort is never enough. We are masters at combining and substituting one drug with another to get high.

Has getting drunk or loaded ever been the unintentional result of "just" one drink or "just" a beer? Have you ever experienced the consequences of impaired judgment or decision-making ability as a direct result of smoking "just" a little pot? Did one of anything ever lead to two or three or more of something harder or stronger?

Many of us never thought that alcohol and/or marijuana were part of our problem, but upon honest examination and working the Steps, we usually find a need to re-evaluate that notion.

PRESCRIPTION DRUGS

The use of prescription drugs may be medically necessary at times. However, old patterns of thinking influenced by the presence of a mind-altering substance in our system can soon have us convinced that we need to take it more frequently than prescribed. An informed prescribing physician, placing our medication in control of someone we can trust, and honest communication with a sponsor or another recovering addict can be helpful in preventing abuse.

Our bodies and minds don't know the difference between drugs used for legitimate reasons and drugs used for recreational pleasure.

It's a sound practice to enlist the support of all of our physicians and/or mental health care professionals in continuing on the path to recovery. Abruptly stopping the use of tranquilizers, antidepressants or other prescription drugs can be dangerous and even deadly, and should only be done under the guidance of an informed physician.

OVER-THE-COUNTER AND COMMONLY USED LEGAL DRUGS

Over-the-counter and other legal drugs (such as cough syrups or pain relievers that contain alcohol and/or codeine, diet pills that act as stimulants, and antihistamines that act as depressants) can be just as big of a problem for us as street drugs. We suggest that you become a label reader. There are many products on the market that can be dangerous to an addict who has the potential to abuse just about any mind-altering chemical.

Uninformed addicts can be a hazard to themselves and others. We encourage you to ask your doctor or pharmacist if you have any questions regarding medications. Be honest with your sponsor about what drugs you take or are prescribed to you.

Remember, we're powerless over cocaine and all other mind-altering substances. Step One is a beginning, but be sure to move forward. A spiritual awakening as the result of working all Twelve Steps is the solution to the problem of addiction.

SO WHAT DOES "... AND ALL OTHER MIND-ALTERING SUBSTANCES" MEAN?

It means that it is the collective experience of the members of Cocaine Anonymous that addiction is a problem not limited to any one substance. It means that C.A.'s Twelve Steps are not drug-specific, and that Cocaine Anonymous is not a drug-specific Fellowship. It means that it doesn't matter to us if you drank or what type of drugs you used; if you have a desire to stop, you are welcome here!

1

OUR HOPE, FAITH AND COURAGE

The early days of Cocaine Anonymous as experienced by two of its members.

When we were asked to write the history of Cocaine Anonymous we were more than pleased, as this was a subject near and dear to us. It is a history that, as a result of timing, good fortune, and grace, we were able to experience first hand. We've had the opportunity to watch an international Fellowship grow up around us with a spirit and enthusiasm that was unfathomable to us some ten years ago.[2]

We were also asked, when writing this story, in the spirit of anonymity, to exclude all names of the players involved; thus placing the focus of this recollection, as well as of this book, on the message rather than on the messengers. The fact of the matter is, that we are all somehow profoundly connected in the pursuit of physical, emotional, and spiritual sobriety. As you read the pages of this book, and hopefully relate and find strength from our experience, you will know in your heart that you, too, have become a part of the history of Cocaine Anonymous.

For the sake of clarity, I would like to explain that there are two of us writing this history. I will refer to us in this story as my partner and I; however, we are much more than that, for we are friends. We had the opportunity a few years ago to conduct a History of C.A. workshop at the World Service Convention in Arizona. We both came to Arizona armed with boxes filled with meeting directories, flyers, tickets, newspaper and magazine clippings, letters, t-shirts, and minutes of business meetings dating back to the beginning of this Fellowship. We sat cross-legged in that elegant

2 This story was originally written for the first C.A. "Storybook," *Hope, Faith & Courage: Stories from the Fellowship of Cocaine Anonymous*, published in 1993. The first meeting of Cocaine Anonymous was held in November 1982.

hotel room, two recovering drug addicts, sorting through papers, swapping stories, laughing and crying about so many events that had chiseled out the course of our lives.

In November 1982, I had been clean and sober for about five months. Prior to that, I had slipped in and out of sobriety in Alcoholics Anonymous for just over a year. I had been a fan in a fellowship where only players grew and thrived. The concept of "being willing to go to any length" was only just then beginning to mean something to me.

One November afternoon, I received a call from a person who had been instrumental in my initial sobriety. This individual, sober for many years already, was calling to inform me of an A.A. meeting at the Motion Picture and Television Fund, in Hollywood, California, that was to take place on the following Tuesday. The topic was to be drugs, especially cocaine. Apparently, the Motion Picture and Television Fund had been flooded with calls from members and others, seeking help for cocaine addiction. Despite the fact that the community at large still considered cocaine to be a nonaddictive drug, there seemed to be an epidemic of nonaddicted, addicted people. I was very excited at the prospect of this meeting. I had been addicted to cocaine, alcohol, pills, psychedelics, opiates, and anything else I could get my hands on. The thought of a forum in which men and women could discuss the solutions of the Twelve Steps and Twelve Traditions in relation to their common experience of bondage to cocaine was most intriguing to me.

The meeting began as does any meeting in Southern California, with the reading of "Chapter Five," from the "Big Book" of Alcoholics Anonymous[3]. It quickly took on an electrifying new dimension. Words like basing, snorting, shooting, copping, scoring,

[3]At the sixth C.A. World Service Conference, held in 1989, a motion was passed to approve the advisory opinion, "The books *Alcoholics Anonymous* and *Twelve Steps and Twelve Traditions* of Alcoholics Anonymous are two of our most valuable tools of recovery and as such, it is the opinion of Cocaine Anonymous that meetings should be allowed to have these books available to support members in their recovery."

dealing, paranoia, and depression went flying around the room with heads nodding and bursts of laughter—our way of expressing the fact that we relate. One member shared about snorting lint from a shag carpet while searching for a rock. Another talked of the desperate feelings of seeing the light come through the corners of the sheets covering the windows, hearing the deafening sound of the morning birds, and of wanting to take his .45 magnum and "waste" those birds; but being afraid to go outside the house because "they" might be out there.

Just prior to the close of this meeting, it was suggested that we take a group conscience to turn this Alcoholics Anonymous meeting into a completely new Twelve-Step program, and call it Cocaine Anonymous. This motion, which sounded like a wonderful idea to me, was quickly voted down. I remember being upset at the time, only to realize later that my thinking had been incorrect; turning an A.A. meeting into a C.A. meeting would have completely disregarded the Twelve Traditions. We would have been trying to turn an apple into an orange. Although they have much in common, they are simply different fruits.

Directly after the meeting that evening, it occurred to a few of us that there was plenty of room and time for both apples and oranges. This was a Tuesday night. We were told by our friend at the Motion Picture and Television Fund that if we returned on Thursday night, there would be a room for us.

Two days later we returned with great anticipation. Approximately twenty members; men and women, newcomers and old-timers from all walks of life, sat in silence at the sound of knuckles hitting the top of a wooden table. A voice I will never forget said, "Welcome to the first Cocaine Anonymous meeting. My name is _____, and I'm an addict and an alcoholic. Cocaine Anonymous is a Fellowship of men and women who share their experience, strength, and hope with each other that they may solve their common problem and help others recover from their addiction." At that moment, you could have heard a pin drop. There was electricity in that room. I believe that as a group, we intuitively knew that something very important had happened, an event that would not just affect our lives, but the lives of countless others for years to come.

At about the same period of time, a hospital in Los Angeles had begun a closed, patient-only meeting, established for addicts whose primary drug was cocaine. Shortly after the inception of Cocaine Anonymous, this hospital meeting opened its doors to all addicts. It became one of the original six Cocaine Anonymous meetings, meetings which seemed to pop up overnight. These became six places a week for cocaine addicts to experience recovery in a safe, supportive environment, where all that was asked of them was to have a desire to be free from their addiction, and to help other addicts achieve the same freedom.

With the existence of these six meetings came the beginning of C.A.'s first attempt to establish a service organization. What this boiled down to was this: each meeting had its secretary represent it at the first service meeting. Given the fact that there were so few of us in attendance, we all miraculously ended up on the Board of Directors. That evening, I made the acquaintance of two other members who were, like myself, driven for some inexplicable reason to devote their next few years to the development and growth of Cocaine Anonymous. Although we were strangers at first and agreed on very little, we quickly developed a strong bond, friendship, and singleness of purpose. Looking back now, I know that we were not being noble; we were simply saving our lives, though none of us realized anything that uncomplicated then.

All three of us, with less than a year of sobriety, along with others, would meet at my house a couple of times a week to discuss, argue, and finally agree on subjects ranging from public information, to literature, to phone lines, to chips, to what to order for dinner that evening. We were starting from scratch, with nothing to lose but our slavery to drugs.

Our first chairperson excelled in his ability to organize. My strong point, as vice-chair, was my ability to motivate and organize others.

My partner, whom I referred to before, was a serious stickler for details. He became the office manager; although, at the time, we didn't actually have an office. We did, however, have a phone and an answering machine. This was our first method used to reach out and be available to addicts who were looking for a meeting, and members around the country who wanted to start meetings in their area.

If you happened to have called in that first year, you would have received a prompt call back from my partner, our office manager. However, chances are, in the first few months of his job, there would have been two people grinding their teeth during that conversation. Unbeknownst to us, my partner was still using periodically, during which time he spoke at length, might I add, and Twelfth-Stepped many people, who years later are still active members.

The phone also became an embarrassment and a lesson to us when we realized that we were compromising the Traditions of C.A.[4] The phone lines were paid for by, and located in, a local drug recovery hospital. We justified this at first, because we were virtually broke, and the phone lines enabled us to reach out. As we began to grow spiritually in our own sobriety, and began to accept guidance from supportive members of Alcoholics Anonymous and Narcotics Anonymous[5], it became all too clear that without our adherence to, and respect for, the Twelve Traditions, we risked the integrity and the very existence of Cocaine Anonymous. We learned we had to be self-supporting through our own contributions, and had to have faith that we would grow accordingly.

There was controversy in those early days that came from those who believed we were unnecessary, that we existed as an "emergency room clearing house" to other fellowships, or that we simply wouldn't survive as a fellowship. We, on the other hand, had read a pamphlet written by the founder of A.A. called *Problems Other*

4 See Appendix C for the Twelve Traditions of Cocaine Anonymous.

5 The Fellowship of Cocaine Anonymous is grateful to individual members of Alcoholics Anonymous (A.A.) and Narcotics Anonymous (N.A.) for their cooperation in our beginning and subsequent survival; however, these references are not meant to imply affiliation.

Than Alcohol, which encouraged us to move forward on our quest and not become part of the controversy. As it turned out, the controversy shortly dissolved into open arms and cooperation from all involved.

It was our hope that the C.A. chips would be a unifying factor in our young Fellowship—something solid to touch, to carry with us, a reminder of our commitment. At that time, we had a hard, white, square chip with letters and numbers. These unfortunately would wear off before you could even get to the next meeting, not to mention that relapsers would use the chips to chop cocaine. In moving to a rounded, more flexible chip, I was asked to come up with three words that would epitomize the spirit of Cocaine Anonymous. Originally, these words were "Hope, Faith and Willingness." Unfortunately, we had to discard the word "Willingness" because it had too many letters. That evening, I sat at home watching a television documentary on President Kennedy. He spoke eloquently on the necessity of having "courage" in our lives. It occurred to me that when many of us walk through the doors of Cocaine Anonymous for the first time, we do so without hope, without faith, but with an ounce of *courage*. We listen to the stories and experiences of others and develop *hope*. As a result of coming back, and coming back, and coming back and working the Twelve Steps, we acquire an abundance of *faith*. Thus were born the guiding principles *Hope, Faith* and *Courage*.

One evening, sitting in an all-night diner with a good friend (whom my partner ironically Twelfth-Stepped, while working the phones "under the influence"), trying to write a suggested standardized meeting format, I found myself deep in discussion about what I believed to be our most pressing obstacle. As women and men came into C.A. they were able, through our fellowship and example, and guidance from the Steps, to give up the use of cocaine, and begin a new life. Unfortunately, many members refused to stop using other substances, explaining that they weren't alcoholics, that pot was a natural herb, or that they really needed those pills to relax or sleep in such a stressful period as early recovery, etc., etc. These members, who usually relapsed on cocaine or began abusing their new drug of choice, often punctuated their case with the challenge, "Anyway, where does it mention anything other than cocaine?" That evening, over a plate of greasy bacon and eggs, we rewrote the First Step, simply adding after the word cocaine: "and all other mind-altering substances"—five little words that almost overnight put to rest this dangerous, life-threatening debate—five little words that told the demons in my head to surrender.

Within a year, the Fellowship had grown to 30 meetings. The days of a handful of us representing the group conscience were over. It was fun while it lasted. But frankly, we were grateful to share the responsibility. For some reason (which eludes me now), the 30 representatives of these 30 meetings decided that we could get more work done if we went on a group service retreat. I still laugh when I think of the chaos and drama that went on between us all; some in our second year, most in their first year, many in their first few months.

The weekend retreat took place at a monastery in the high desert. Respecting the monks' traditions, we ate breakfast in silence. But we never stopped bickering the rest of the day. Like so many other challenges we were meeting in our new clean and sober lives, by the end of this weekend we had developed a sense of community and a feeling of unity.

The weekend ended with a C.A. meeting in the monks' cemetery at the close of a clear, beautiful day. We each took our turn, sharing our gratitude and love, as the sun began to set and a cold wind blew across the desert floor. Suddenly, interrupting a particularly heartfelt share, one of the representatives (with three months off freebase) reached into his pocket and cried out, "Oh no!" He pulled out a rather large plastic bag filled with cocaine. Thirty hearts began to race. Thirty minds began to run. As a group, we simply froze. The thought of the entire service structure of C.A. being wiped out in an afternoon was too absurd. Someone nervously suggested we take a group conscience. Another member jokingly proposed we sell the blow and donate the profits. Before this event got too out of hand, before the sun set altogether beyond the horizon, with the last bits of light shooting across the desert, a large gust of wind arose. This wise newcomer opened the bag, grabbed the bottom, and began to wave it in the air. In a moment, a cloud of white powder went floating away into the twilight. We sat there as a group in silence, as if we were saying goodbye to an old friend. We were in awe at the knowledge that together, with the help of a Higher Power, we could do what individually had always eluded us. We held hands, said the Serenity Prayer, and went home.

During the next two and one-half years, C.A. grew at a remarkable rate. As the result of articles about "the cocaine epidemic and recovery" that mentioned Cocaine Anonymous in the *Los Angeles Times, People, Time,* and *Newsweek*, inquiries about the program began to flow in. We were overwhelmed by this response. It became apparent to us, especially my partner, that the time for a world service organization had arrived. Our amazing growth in California was paralleled by C.A. fellowships cropping up in several cities throughout the United States.

Within this time period, we received an envelope from the Chicago Fellowship that contained a pamphlet they had written and were offering for our consideration, in hopes it would become C.A.'s first piece of literature. We, in the California contingency, had been working very hard on a piece already. But between us, we couldn't agree on a single page. With tremendous skepticism, we sat and read aloud this bold offering from this far away place. It was perfect. With mouths hanging open and tears in our eyes, we knew that these words said exactly what needed to be said. It was entitled *To the Newcomer* and includes what is now referred to as *Who is a Cocaine Addict?,* which is read aloud at many meetings throughout the world.

On May 3, 1985, hundreds of recovering addicts converged on a beachfront hotel in Santa Barbara, California, to attend the first annual World Service Convention. It was called the Seaside Unity and Acceptance Convention, but was much, much more than that. Voices from the phone and names from letters were taking form. Faces of old friends we had not as yet met appeared there before us. From coast to coast we came—excited, curious and filled with an energy that was to become our trademark.

In a crowded room on a Saturday morning, the diligent chairperson of World Services cautiously called to order the first national business meeting. After a passionate exchange of ideas, which set the format for future conferences, the meeting came to a close with a remarkable feeling of optimism.

That night we gathered together in the hotel's banquet hall to feast and celebrate our new Fellowship. Men and women who had only recently graced bathrooms, prisons, mental wards, and treatment centers were now seated in this balloon-filled majestic room, shoulder-to-shoulder, looking and feeling alive and well. The speaker was inspiring to our already high-spirited group. Banquet food even seemed to taste good that night. The first chairperson, and my partner and I were recognized that evening as C.A.'s first Trustees. This recognition somehow represented to us, and to those present, the spiritual connection and acceptance of what was, and what could be in the future. The highlight of the evening was the state-by-state countdown. One by one, each participating state was announced. Its representatives rose to the cheers and applause that grew to a fevered pitch, as voices cried out: "Alaska, Arizona, California, Connecticut, District of Columbia, Georgia, Hawaii, Illinois, Nevada, New Jersey, New York, Ohio, Tennessee, Texas, Virginia, Washington, and Wisconsin."

In the years since that convention, C.A. has spread its message and enthusiasm throughout the United States, beyond the border to Canada, and across the Atlantic Ocean to Europe.[6]

[6] The Cocaine Anonymous World Service Office has received requests for Meeting Starter Kits from around the world.

When I was newly sober it was explained to me that the Greek definition of the word "enthusiasm" is, "en," meaning "in" or "with," and "theos" meaning "God." In other words—having God within. One day at a time, the Fellowship of Cocaine Anonymous enthusiastically carries the message of Cocaine Anonymous throughout the world to the addict who has the courage to ask for help.

A while back, I had a most disturbing dream. It began like a retrospective collage, covering my clean and sober years. I dreamt of friends and lovers whose wisdom had altered my damaged way of thinking, of events like those covered in this story: the wonder of the first C.A. meeting and the excitement of the Seaside Unity and Acceptance Convention. I dreamt of working the Steps and experiencing a new sense of well-being, blended perfectly with a rebirth of my passion. I dreamt of courage, hope, and faith, of learning that "success may be getting what you want, but happiness is wanting what you get."

All at once, in a flash, I dreamt that I awoke. Still dreaming, I believed that all my clean and sober years had never happened. That I was again "coming to" that day, still caught in the horrifying grips of a progressive state of high anxiety, loneliness, despair, and addiction. My body filled with spasms, my mind with paranoia, my spirit deadened; I was pathetic. These thoughts hurled me into a state of panic.

I broke out in a sweat, my eyes flew open, and at last I was awake, for real. Still groggy and frightened, I shook as I tried to remember what was true. Slowly but surely, I took a deep breath, got into the moment and knew that everything was as it should be; I wasn't alone. I was clean and sober; I had experienced a complete psychic change; I was safe.

Suddenly, I was overcome with a clear euphoric sensation, as I intuitively understood that even if the nightmare had been true, even if I was still back in the land of hopelessness, chances are I might still find help. All at once, I had the revelation that what I would have to do is get out of bed, get dressed, find another addict with the courage to change, and tell him about my dream.

2

EAP TO C.A. AND HP TO LIFE

Her most life-changing moment of all was when her boss sent her to the Employee Assistance Program that began the path of living in recovery.

I grew up in the 1950s, a post-World-War-II baby. I was an only child until my brother came along when I was three. I was the favorite of the grandchildren, and I knew it. Being the oldest usually meant I got the most, the biggest, and the best of what there was to offer the kids. Despite this obvious abundance, I never really felt adequate among family or friends.

Among my friends, I was the one who always had the allowance, clothes, toys, games, and everything else I wanted. I used it to my advantage, to pay for movies or meals, buy my friends presents, and basically be the most independent in the group. The addictive behavior was already there as I bought friends and lovers and sold myself in the process.

When I was in high school and during my first two years at the local junior college, I was totally anti-marijuana. I practically campaigned against it to my friends, telling them how terrible one's life would become under the influence of pot and the other drugs marijuana would surely lead to. I quoted the health book where I got all my information; I was staunch about this and made no secret about my opinions.

Then one weekend I attended a "sleep in your car or sleep in the mud, but just sleep with someone" rock concert, where I witnessed some kids smoking a joint. I didn't realize it at the time, but this small incident changed my life.

I returned to college more aware of the language and lifestyles of these "drug users." I began to understand some of the phrases that previously had gone over my head. Within months, I was smoking pot with my younger brother, who had been doing so without my knowledge for quite some time. I spent the next two years in college smoking pot and swallowing pills. I finally felt like I was really a part of the cool crowd. Life was good, and I was a part of it.

I graduated from college and became a teacher. I smoked once in a while and drank a lot. It was easy to enjoy drinking wine; ladies drank wine, and I was a lady. Drinking also enabled me to meet and become involved with many men. I spent two years in that town smoking pot, taking pills, sleeping with lots of men, and eating to make myself feel better about whatever I didn't want to feel. I still thought life was good.

I took a year off and moved to another state. During that year, I was introduced to cocaine. I loved it! I began snorting it all the time, and since I could afford to buy it, I always had it handy. I moved back to my city and got a job here. There was always an abundance of pills, powder, discos, men, food, and parties. This went on for a few years, and I had it all under control. I didn't eat too much; I didn't use too much cocaine or take too many pills; I didn't think that I slept with too many men. Then, in the early 1980s, someone showed me how to smoke cocaine. We called it freebase. I loved the ritual and the process, the sneaky ways we bought it, prepared it, and smoked it.

Around this time, my grandfather, with whom I was extremely close, passed away. This man was my idol. He had been the only relative who never criticized or corrected me; he seemed to love me when I didn't feel like I got love from anyone else. His death caused a hole in my heart that seemed unfillable. One night during that week of mourning, I was freebasing, and I got a feeling unlike anything I had ever experienced. All the pain and inadequacy went away that night.

In the weeks and months that followed, the frequency with which I continued to get high was unlike anything in the past. I didn't want to feel anything except that ringing in my ears and the euphoria that followed. I was on my way. I spent entire nights smoking; I brought cocaine to my job and smoked it on my breaks; I missed appointments; I stopped paying bills; I wouldn't answer the telephone when collectors called; I no longer spent time with my friends and very little with my relatives, but I still thought I was enjoying myself.

I had sent the live-in boyfriend packing when I learned to cop, cook, and smoke freebase without his help. Once during an argument, he called me a junkie. How dare he! I knew he was wrong. Junkies were those filthy street people who stuck dirty heroin-filled needles in their arms, and I certainly wasn't one of them! How ironic that even the man who had shown me how to use the stuff was worried that I used too much and would soon be dead. I was slowly becoming a suicide statistic, yet I still thought my life was so good.

By 1985, I was in so much pain, emotionally and physically, that I was no longer thinking life was so good. Money was running out, and I was completely in debt. My close friends were making other plans, and my family could not understand why I never showed up on time, if at all. I had scabs covering my body and sores from compulsively picking at them. Finally, my boss sent me to the Employee Assistance Program (EAP) for the help I knew I needed but was unable to ask for.

All these years later, I still thank my Higher Power for the greatest life-changing moment of all. I'm convinced it was with divine intervention that my boss changed the course of my life. Drugs were about to ruin my career. The EAP counselor talked to me about the drug use and how I needed to stop right now. I admitted to her that I had a little problem and said that I would try to stop. By then I had unsuccessfully tried to stop a couple of times. Somewhere in the fog in my head, I heard her mention something about "packing a bag." In that instant, I was jolted into a life-changing moment of reality.

Things happened quickly during the next several days and I entered a 28-day treatment facility. To this day, I can recall the receptionist telling me on the phone, "No one here will hurt you." She was right.

On my first night in treatment, I had sex on the floor of the meeting room with one of the men there. My life had become so unmanageable that I thought that was normal. During my first few days in treatment, I sat on the floor instead of a chair because I was so used to sitting that way in my home with my pipe. I didn't want to be there, but I didn't want to go home. I saw the list of Twelve Steps posted on the wall, and I could not relate. During the days, I contributed very little to the group. At night, I attended Twelve-Step meetings and watched as people came in smiling, sat in chairs, and read pieces of literature about drug and alcohol addiction. I listened as some of them told their stories or shared their feelings about their new lives without drugs. I didn't understand fully, so I just sat in the back row, and when it was over, I went to bed. This went on for a few days.

My counselor talked to me about the Twelve Steps of recovery. It took me a while to understand that I had a disease and that recovery was possible, and that it would take some work and I would need to be willing to follow directions. He told me that the answer was in those Twelve Steps on the wall, and I began to pay attention.

My head began to clear a bit, and I could actually see myself getting clean. I began to work the Steps. I wrote pages about not only the fact that I was powerless over my addictions, but that my life had become unmanageable. How manageable had it been to arrive late to school more than 47 days in one school year and scream at the custodians when I was unable to open the locked door? How manageable had it been to write bad checks for department store gift certificates, then spend hours searching for the "right" $3 item so as not to waste the cash I got back from the certificate so I could go buy cocaine?

I wrote on the Second Step and shared with my group how I had come to believe that a Power greater than myself could restore me to sanity. I had a lifetime of insane experiences centered on how I felt inadequate and unloved. I was finally coming to believe that I didn't have to think that way anymore. All this was coming along quite nicely—and then came the Third Step.

I had always been independent, self-reliant, and financially secure. Now I was expected to turn my will and my life over to a Power greater than myself. I struggled with this for days. How could it be that someone like me who had college degrees, money, brains, and status should be expected to stop trying to control my own life and allow someone else to do it? This was hard for me, but I was beginning to learn about willingness and God. I prayed and waited. Finally, I understood that this Step was asking me to turn my will and my life over to "the care" of God. This was something I could do. It became clear that just like the "day at a time" concept of the program, these Steps are written so that we can take each Step, and each part of the Step, a little bit at a time, so it won't be painfully overwhelming.

I was told that I needed to begin writing my Fourth Step before leaving treatment. I began writing about my resentments, my fears, and my sexual activities. I didn't fully understand exactly why I was writing it all, but by this time, I was willing to take direction because I believed that it would help me. It did.

After being in the facility for 28 days, it was time to leave, and I didn't want to go home. I had grown to love the warmth and safety of the treatment center, and I was afraid of what I would face back home and in the world. My father came for me, but before we left, I had one more thing to do. I had become friendly with one of the nurses, and I asked her to be my sponsor.

I went home and got back into my life. I called my sponsor every day. I continued to write my Fourth Step, and after a few months, I was ready to share it with her.

While all this was going on, I was still attending aftercare twice weekly. One day, my counselor handed me a starter kit for a Fellowship called Cocaine Anonymous, which was already growing throughout the country but had no meetings where I lived. About a dozen of us began that first meeting when I had 89 days clean. I was unaware at the time that this was to be another life-changing moment for me. I did not relate to alcohol or other drugs as well as

I did to cocaine. Even though none of us had ever been to a C.A. meeting, we all felt at home there, and the meetings began to multiply, first in the local vicinity, then in the state.

I have been involved in service work for Cocaine Anonymous ever since. I feel more connected in Cocaine Anonymous, and it is for that reason that I stay. Since that first meeting, there are now dozens of C.A. meetings across our state with hundreds of recovering addicts getting and carrying the message of recovery. I have even been fortunate in being involved in online meetings of Cocaine Anonymous—yes, there are actually C.A. meetings on the internet for addicts who are unable to get to face-to-face meetings.

As the years went by, I remained in service work and an active member of Cocaine Anonymous. I can't say that my program was a perfect one; I have made mistakes. When I was clean and sober for seven years, I became involved with a man who was good-looking and sexy—and HIV positive. When I was with him, my old feelings of inadequacy surfaced. I spent lots of money on him and allowed him to take full advantage of me, including sexually, even though I was aware of his diagnosis. Dating him made me feel "normal" and part of the crowd, just as the drugs had so many years before. As a consequence of that relationship, today I am HIV positive.

Ironically, the former live-in boyfriend who had called me a junkie had turned his own life around and had become an HIV/AIDS counselor. It was he who shared the diagnosis information with me. In many ways, that diagnosis was one of the best things to have ever happened to me. It took me a while, but over the years, I have developed an appreciation for life and health that I never had before.

I have learned that if I don't continue to work on my defects of character on a daily basis, my program and possibly my life will be in jeopardy. I have made many of the amends on my list, and when the opportunities come, I make more. I thank God every morning for the chance to breathe one more day, and I thank Him again at night. I realize on a daily basis how imperfect I am, and for this, I am grateful for that Tenth Step. I am learning to meditate, and I seek to know what God's will is for me. I have come to know that He wants nothing bad for His children. It is this comforting thought that sustains me much of the time. I go to meetings and continue to carry the message of Cocaine Anonymous and recovery. I have a sponsor, the same woman whom I asked on that day when I had 28 days clean. I have sponsees scattered around the globe and the internet, who I am honored to know and grateful to call my friends. I converse daily with my Higher Power, without my faith in Whom none of this could have happened.

My recovery has taken me to places around the globe I never dreamed of seeing. Being clean and sober has given me the opportunities to meet many loving and wonderful people all over the world. I have enjoyed moments and memories in recovery that I would have never been alive to witness or experience without sobriety and the program of Cocaine Anonymous in my life.

3

READY FOR ANYTHING

She was looking for help to get rid of a drug problem, but what she found was an entire new way of life.

I am a cocaine addict. I love to hear myself say that. Today I am grateful to be a cocaine addict. Cocaine taught me something that I needed to learn, and I doubt I would have ever learned it without cocaine.

I didn't try pot until I was in my early thirties. I never liked booze and only drank when I couldn't refuse the obligatory glass of champagne at some formal occasion. I didn't like the taste of alcoholic drinks, and, more important, I hated the light feeling in my head. I feared losing control and being embarrassed because under the influence I would do or say things that I normally wouldn't.

Looking back, I see now that control was very important in my life. I was a very shy kid, bullied at primary school, and raised in a family where verbal abuse and aggression were standard. There was a lot of fear. I was always looking for ways to change the mood of the people around me, to prevent them from being angry or to make myself invisible. I didn't feel safe or comfortable, and I tried to find ways to change the things around me that I feared. When I could, I tried to create a safe space to hide.

I was the second of three daughters. My sisters constantly argued with one another and with my parents. I took on the role of the good kid, trying to comfort my mother, who suffered the most and used me for emotional comfort. I was intelligent and performed well at school, so at school I was the smart kid. The kids with whom I socialized were like that, too; we looked down on people who got drunk and smoked cigarettes, let alone smoked pot—anything heavier was beyond our imagination.

I left high school the year my parents divorced. I went to university to study theology and found life quite overwhelming. I had survived the school system despite hating it, and told myself I was free at last. I was free from living with parents that were obsessed with fighting each other, but I didn't feel free.

I got my first boyfriend and had my first sexual experiences. My idea of a relationship was to have as much sex as possible, trying to squeeze the rest of life (study, jobs, house, family, friends) into as little time as possible. Most of my life revolved completely about my boyfriend. I quit my studies but didn't have a job. I didn't bother to pay attention to my life and my responsibilities. My life was too messed up to deal with, so all that mattered was his job, his family, and his problems.

Meanwhile, I expected my boyfriend to take care of me, make sense of my life, and be available for me when I had emotional problems 24/7. I felt mostly depressed and hopeless about my situation, but I pushed those feelings aside.

After a while I got involved with someone else. I had numerous relationships and affairs. I was looking for the miracle, wrapped in a man, which would make my life worthwhile and make me feel like a real person. I began to combine pot and sex. I liked it, and although it seemed to be a great discovery, after a while I wanted more.

I started to act out a lot of my fantasies, only to feel cheap and abused. To compensate for that, I started to ask for money for sex. Being a prostitute was one of my oldest fantasies, and it gave me the sense of power and security that I had always longed for.

I was introduced to cocaine by one of my dates. I liked it, especially the sexual rush it gave me. I started dating a cocaine dealer and soon was introduced to freebasing. I was hooked from my first hit. It crossed my mind for a split second that there would be no going back from that point, but I did it anyway. I immediately stopped being interested in snorting, and I stopped trying to control my using after a few times of smoking freebase. I found I couldn't stop, and trying to stop spoiled the whole enterprise, so when I did it, I did it good. That pipe made me feel how I was supposed to feel.

All my problems, insecurity, inhibitions, and fears were not just gone—it was as if they had never existed.

I had my own business and worked as a contractor. I only used on weekends, maybe twice a month, but I got worried because of the effect it had on me even when I was not using. When I started thinking about using, it drove me nuts; the thoughts were all-consuming. I went to the local drug counseling agency, and they told me that it was dangerous and I should never do it again, but they couldn't tell me if I was an addict or what an addict was. My boyfriend, the dealer, told me there was nothing wrong with what we were doing. Since he was more into the habit than I was, and he wasn't an addict, that reassured me. Besides that, all the agency could offer me was to take a hot shower when I felt the urge to use, so there was little help to be expected from them.

I thought I should seek some professional help for my depression and maybe that would help me to not use so often. But I stopped going after I found I could lie or smart talk about my cocaine use without being asked any further questions.

When I started to use almost every weekend, I made a resolution to stop. When I couldn't go to work and called in sick one Monday morning, I made a resolution to stop. When I started to pay for the dope myself because we'd smoked all the stock and the profit, I made a resolution to stop. When I thought my boyfriend had died of an overdose while he was having an epileptic seizure, I made a resolution to stop. When I started to use at my own house, I made a resolution to stop. When I used after I had made a resolution to stop, I made another resolution to stop.

I was living a triple life, and I got more worried. My family, with whom I wasn't close, didn't know about any of this. No one knew about the cocaine. On Monday morning, I couldn't honestly remember anything about the weekend because I was leading different lives which were completely disconnected.

Whenever I had a moment on my own, I was depressed and lonely. I was very negative and cynical about life in general, hopeless about my life in particular, and in denial about all of this. I think I perceived myself as numb and exhausted, in denial one day at a time. Another part of me indulged in suicidal fantasies, although I had already concluded years ago that I was too much of a coward to face an unsuccessful attempt. Yet, whenever I had a conscious moment, the most positive thought I had was a desire to die in my sleep.

While internet surfing on a new computer, I came across an article about cocaine. Obsessed as I was with my favorite candy, a few links later I was on the C.A. website. I was unfamiliar with any Twelve-Step program or Fellowship and felt funny about the "anonymous" part. I wondered if maybe these people had the secret of how to use and not go insane. I took the self-test and was convinced I was an addict. It all made too much sense for comfort. My lies and denial were punctured without me knowing they were lies or even the meaning of the word "denial."

I decided I was going to quit for real. Although I had always vowed I could stop if I wanted to and that I would stop if I were an addict, I knew that quitting for real was going to be very seriously tough. I made an inquiry and found C.A. didn't exist in my country. I was turned off by the Higher Power stuff, which I thought to be sentimental B.S., but I was going to try to quit. I had to because I didn't want to be an addict.

I did quit, white-knuckling and with all I had in me. It lasted eight weeks.

I was devastated when I used again, and it wasn't even as good as it always had been. I knew I was done. I knew I was going to quit again, and I knew I was going to get loaded again. I would quit and get loaded again, then quit again and get loaded again. That cycle would be repeated over and over. I knew I wanted to stop, but I knew there was nothing in me that could make me stay stopped.

I told myself I had tried everything, but I was a very good liar, and I believed most of my lies because I told so many of them that I had lost the truth a long time ago. At that moment, I knew I couldn't tell myself any more lies. I was done.

Completely numb, I started to repair my computer, which had broken. I needed some distraction because I knew if I were to face the truth, I would break into so many pieces that I would be completely lost. I couldn't allow myself to face the despair and the loss of all perspective. It was too dark, too scary, and too real. I wanted it to not be real, but I knew it was, and I did not know how to face up to the reality I had created.

When I got my computer working again, I found an e-mail from the C.A. helpline. The person wondered how I was doing after we had corresponded about cocaine addiction and my resolution to stop. The message ended with, "Are you still clean? Great!! Did you get loaded? Just dust yourself off and start again." I broke down in tears. No "I told you so" or anything. That acceptance made me believe that I could accept myself and my situation.

I cried my heart out and e-mailed back what had happened. I received a very brief response that ended with, "Are you ready to take serious Steps?" I replied I was. I had no clue what that meant, but from the depths of my despair, I knew I was ready to do anything to get out of this. Not only was the path that I saw ahead of me a hopeless fight against cocaine that I knew I was going to lose, I had also lost the one and only comfort that freed me from the depression and lack of direction. My only friend had turned into a mean and overpowering enemy, and I had to face the miserable and terrifying state of my life without any escape now.

I was ready for anything, even if it could save me for only one day. I was almost certain I would fail, but anything was better than trying to find hope in my worn-out, fake attempts. I was overwhelmed that someone would reach out to the messy, dirty wreck that I was, full of shame and guilt, and that someone had some hope for me.

I received three directions: to pray every day, to keep in touch for 90 days in a row while being completely honest, especially about my feelings, and to not use today. I felt an enormous relief at how easy and do-able these tasks were.

I started and completed working the Steps with this person, who became my first sponsor. I have not had an urge to use since. I didn't understand much of what I was doing, and I certainly disliked and or feared most of it, but I did it. I was often driven only by the motivation to prove my sponsor wrong. Everything I tried, hoping to find it didn't work for me so I could stop, did work.

I joined online meetings and started going to face-to-face meetings. When I couldn't find any literature, people from online meetings sent some to me. I started to read. After a couple of weeks, I remember looking forward to coming home after work because I was going to work my Steps.

For the first time in a great number of years, I felt I was doing something that actually made sense. Positive little things started to enter my life, from the first days and weeks of recovery. I was very happy counting days that I woke up and went to bed clean. I was amazed at how much I could relate to what I was reading. It was not all uplifting, but I was very happy to finally understand something about myself, to have a frame in which all of me fit. I saw that the disease had always been there, and everything started to make sense.

Today my life has undergone an immense change. I am no longer depressed, not even when it is autumn and dark, grey weather is approaching. I am happy and grateful to be alive. I am okay with myself. Even when the circumstances are not okay, I am still okay. That is a 180-degree difference from my prior view of life. Before, I had always thought the whole world around me (including wars and disasters) had to be okay before I would be able to feel okay. Today I can accept my emotions. I can take responsibility for my life and make choices. I learned to stand up for my boundaries. I learned to take care of my needs and to take care of myself. I have a spiritual life for the first time.

I am learning how to behave in a healthy relationship. I thought I had screwed up so much that I could never be involved in a close personal relationship again. Now I have experienced love—unconditional love. I know the difference between self-pity and pain.

I learned to identify, accept, and face my fears, and a Power greater than myself has been there to help me walk through it every time.

I was looking for help to get rid of a drug problem, but what I found is an entire new way of life. I always thought I was cool, but I was lacking direction long before I started doing cocaine. I am now convinced there was no other way. Cocaine brought me to where I needed to be: on my knees. The Higher Power that I found through the Twelve Steps is showing me what my life is really about.

Through all the insanity and obsessions, I was always looking for spiritual answers. I tried so many things—like yoga, meditation, reiki, astrology, self-help stuff, New Age and ancient philosophies—always looking for the meaning of life and an answer for my problems but never giving myself to anything. The Twelve Steps not only showed me a way out of the prison of self-justification and destructive obsessions, they have the answer to my deepest questions in a way that I can understand and practice. I was always doing the spiritual talk, but today I am shown a spiritual path I can walk, one little step at a time.

I finally have a goal in life that answers all my questions. I know I don't need to arrive at the goal before I can start living, but I have a direction for every next step I take. The goal in my life today is to be of service to my Higher Power and to others. Where the root of my disease is to be self-centered, the solution is that I can help myself through helping others—or my Higher Power can reach out to me and help me when I reach out to others and dedicate myself to helping them. That is something I can practice every day. I don't need money, education, people, books, diplomas, positions, power, or any resources other than my own time and willingness. My willingness comes from a deep, deep sense of gratitude that I have been helped to escape living a slow death.

I flew to the U.S.A. to do my Fifth Step when I was a couple of months clean. I was given a meeting starter kit and was involved with the first C.A. meeting in my country. Since then, we have grown to six meetings. I have also been connected to C.A. through conventions and online meetings that were very, very important to me. There I was surrounded by people for whom relapse was simply not an option, and I just copied what they did. I developed a passion for carrying the message via Hospitals and Institutions and Public Information (H&I and PI) because I know there are many others like me who are worried and have no clue C.A. is here. Being involved in service and working the Steps with a bunch of women is absolutely vital to my recovery. It is the quickest and easiest way out of myself, out of my disease. The Twelve Steps make me ready for the real solution: to be of service in a healthy way. Helping others is the way to both help myself and to grow into another person.

What seemed to be completely, utterly, a hundred percent impossible is not really hard today. The Steps changed me into someone who doesn't need cocaine to endure or master life. Life is okay. My life is okay. Even when everything in my life is not okay, it is still okay to be me, to be alive. Some people say they are happy because they have their old life back. I am happy because my old life died, and I hope it will never be returned to me. My Higher Power has given me an entire new chance to live.

4

SET FREE BY THE TRUTH

After being released from jail, he was still imprisoned by secrets about his addiction. Getting honest was his key to freedom.

I was raised in an alcoholic household where I learned to manipulate, lie, cheat, steal, and especially to disappear when things were going bad. I also learned to be a peacemaker, a people pleaser, and to smile in the face of disaster. As a child I always felt afraid, less than, ashamed, guilty, and humiliated.

One weekend when I was 12 years old, I was suddenly introduced to a number of different drugs. Somewhere in that combination of chemicals, I found my answer. I was no longer afraid. I was no longer ashamed. I no longer felt less than. I did not care about guilt. I also did not see any line to cross, no long hard road leading to addiction. I believed I had found the missing piece that completed the picture of my life. I would spend the next 20 years trying to duplicate the feeling I found that weekend.

Very early during those years, I learned to use violence and intimidation so that no one would know I was afraid. I went into every situation with an attitude. In high school, I got into many fights and a lot of trouble. Soon, I was not welcome in school, so I dropped out, took my graduate equivalency degree, and began my history of geographic changes. I always thought I was running "to" something. It was years later before I realized I was actually running from my own fears.

My first geographic change was to join the United States Navy. My naval career was disastrous. I got two women pregnant overseas, smuggled drugs, and ended my tour early with a felony conviction for international transportation of narcotics. However, the military had been given a new option to use for drug convictions, and the Navy was willing to try it out on me. So I got a huge break and served a minimal amount of time in federal prison, attended a drug treatment program, and was given an "Other than Honorable" discharge.

I went home for a while, but I was uncomfortable under the watchful eyes of my family, so I ran off to another state. Within a year, I had lost a lot of weight and all of my material possessions and was living on the streets of a large city. I was panhandling and stealing to supply my dope habit and to eat on those rare occasions when I wasn't high. Around Thanksgiving, I got on a Greyhound bus headed home. My parents met me about 150 miles away from home to check me into another treatment center. After 30 days in treatment, I went back to live in my parents' house.

I stayed clean for a while, entered college, and got married. Right from the start, my wife and I were always looking for that greener pasture. I began using not long after the marriage and soon was using just like the "old days." My wife and I were fighting all the time, and I was staying out until all hours of the night. My violence became directed at myself in the form of suicide attempts. My wife started seeking companionship elsewhere. One night I caught her at an old boyfriend's house, and I knew we were through.

I went home, drank down some illicit prescription drugs with some liquor, and locked her out of the house. My soon-to-be-ex-wife called the cops. The night ended with me going to jail for aggravated assault on a police officer and her going back to her high school sweetheart.

I served part of my sentence in the prison psych ward where I was diagnosed as bipolar with violent tendencies. The prison doctor told me that my drug use was an attempt to self-medicate, but that it would always end in a violent episode.

While I was locked up, I was introduced to a lovely young lady through a mutual friend. We wrote each other for the next year while I served out my time in prison. This was the first time in my life I got to know a woman before I jumped into bed with her. When I was released, I moved in with this woman, and we began our life together. Unfortunately, our addictions came with us. We got married, had two sons, and managed for a while. We moved to "make things better." I did another short stint in a county jail for distribution of a controlled substance.

Finally, however, my addiction took over, and I became the person I was always afraid of being—someone my family was scared to be around. My wife kicked me out of the house. I tried suicide, went to the psych ward, and then she let me move back in. After a few weeks, she kicked me out again, and the vicious cycle continued.

One desperate night, I went by the house and found one of my drug acquaintances in bed with my wife, getting her high with dope he had stolen from me. In my violent rage, I almost killed this man, and I brutalized and attempted to rape the woman I love. It seemed the prison doctor was right: my addiction always took me to that dark, violent place.

I was arrested but allowed to post bail. I went on the run. I was living on the streets, stealing a lot and panhandling a little, always looking over my shoulder. By the time the police caught me, new charges had been added, and I was off to prison again.

One morning as I sat in my cell, I realized it was Thanksgiving. I wondered if anyone knew where I was or if they even cared. I had disregarded the feelings of everyone who had ever loved me, including myself. I was filled with shame, guilt, and remorse. I felt all the pain of all those years rush through me. I felt all the shame for my deeds and humiliation for what I had become. In that instant I truly felt all the despair of a dying man. I looked up and said, "God, if you even exist, end this all now. I want to die."

I believe my Higher Power has a warped sense of humor, for just as I finished my first honest prayer, the jailer came in and said, "There is a meeting about to start. Any takers?"

I was furious! I had been in and out of a Twelve-Step program for years and had stayed loaded. I was convinced that the program didn't work. I decided now to prove it to everyone else. So I went to the meeting which was brought in by a Hospitals and Institutions (H&I) Committee. By the time the meeting was over, I was committed to doing all the things they suggested—just to prove that the program didn't work.

I immediately began working the Steps and going to the meetings that were available in the prison. Slowly my attitude started to change. Surprisingly, I began to believe that there might be hope for me yet.

Divorce papers were delivered. I wanted to use drugs to cover the pain, but words from the H&I meetings kept coming back to me: "You can't do this for anyone but yourself."

My ex-wife began to bring my sons to see me in prison. I found out she had started going to Cocaine Anonymous after that last terrifying night. Gradually, we started talking. Eventually we made some much-needed amends.

At 18 months sober, I was working on a Fourth Step when I got locked down for 30 days with a heroin user who was getting almost daily shipments under our door. After 21 days, I finally cracked and used. I felt the drug hit me, and then I thought, "Oh, my God—what did I just do?" I climbed up on my bunk, covered my head with the blanket, and wanted to die. I didn't tell anyone of my relapse.

When I was released, I returned to my ex-wife. I got involved with Cocaine Anonymous, found a sponsor, and started working with him. I worked the Twelve Steps, became of service to C.A., and was very active in the groups, business meetings, and committees, especially H&I.

Things began to work in my life despite myself. My ex-wife and I remarried, surrounded by all our friends in the program. My kids were no longer afraid of me. I had begun a loving relationship with my family again. I was able to hold down a job. I had started using solutions in my life that weren't violent or abusive. I tried to develop a conscious contact with a Higher Power.

There was only one problem. I hadn't been completely honest, and the secret was eating me alive. I was coming up on what everyone believed was my fourth sobriety birthday when I realized I could no longer live the lie. I told my sponsor about the day in prison when I used. He said, "There will come a time when the only thing standing between you and the next drug or drink will be a conscious contact with a Higher Power. Did you have a conscious contact that day?"

"No," I said. I also discovered that the shame, guilt, and humiliation of my secret had blocked me from connecting with a Higher Power. I began working the Steps again with my sponsor.

I was afraid to admit my secret, but I was even more afraid of using and dying. So I set out to tell everyone the truth, believing that I was about to lose my family, my friends, the Fellowship, and that I was going to be humiliated, shamed, and belittled.

I could not have been more wrong. I experienced more love and understanding than I ever thought possible. It was a humbling and spiritual experience. I began to believe that God would do for me what I could not do myself. Life has always been rather baffling to me, but today I walk through life with my Higher Power.

Today I can love myself and look in the mirror without wanting to cry or hang my head in shame for the things I have done. Cocaine Anonymous and my Higher Power have helped me to become someone my family and friends can trust. Today I can love my family the way the program has taught me—unconditionally. My mother no longer has dreams of me dying of an overdose. I can talk with my father and brother again. I also have a program family that has always given me a hand up and taught me to repay each kindness by giving someone else a hand up.

My wife and I remain active in Cocaine Anonymous, especially with H&I. I have been taught about forgiveness and about participating in my own recovery by cleaning my side of the street. In meetings and with H&I, I share my experience, strength, and hope so that another addict might hear the message that finally brings them home. I meet with my sponsor and sponsees on a regular basis to work on the Steps and do what is necessary to keep this freedom that I have been given.

There is an old joke about a country-western song where the man loses everything—relationship, friends, house, job, truck, even his dog. But when the record is played backwards, he gets everything back. During my active addiction, I lost my family, friends, house, conscience, and my soul. My Higher Power has played the record of my life backwards, and I have been given all of these things back, and more.

5

DERAILED

His life was a train wreck. Now he's living the dream.

My life had become a complete train wreck. I sat alone in a hotel room. In front of me were a half-empty bottle of whiskey, a half-empty vial of cocaine, and a fully loaded .44 revolver. I wasn't sure which I was going to put to my head. For reasons I don't fully understand today, but which I accept to be the work of my Higher Power, I didn't feel it necessary to use any of those deadly options that night, and haven't since.

Today, looking back over my life, I believe that I was born with the potential to be an alcoholic and addict. All I ever wanted was to feel loved and cared for, to feel a part of, to feel comfortable, but it always seemed like I was on the outside looking in. I was uncomfortable in my own skin. Somehow, being me just never seemed good enough.

Objectively, I had it pretty good. Subjectively, I felt I was grossly inadequate and couldn't measure up. I had a loving family, a ton of friends, everything I needed, and yet I felt lousy about everything. My life was great, but because my perceptions were distorted, I didn't see it that way.

I spent the greater portion of my life searching for something to plug into those empty holes in my soul, one by one, just to get through the day. I continually changed my personality to blend in with my background.

As I found out many years later, the bottom line was that my disease was the problem. You see, I got the "ism," and it's inside me where the madness lies. No matter where I run, no matter where I hide, no matter what mask I put on, eventually whatever's inside me rises to the surface and rears its ugly little head.

I was soul-sick and lost. I started gambling as a kid, acting out violently as an early teen, and drinking in my middle teens. The effect these actions produced in my mind was astonishing. I was somehow able to feel on the inside the way you looked on the outside.

As the result of my chameleon-like persona, I did well in school. I was a college athlete, president of the university's interfraternity council, and I married my high school sweetheart. I eventually owned real estate and businesses, and I was successful and wealthy by my mid-twenties. I worked hard and I played hard, but the party train finally began taking its toll.

Although I was the last to see it, there were obvious signs of unmanageability sprouting up throughout my life. I wasn't spending very much time with my wife anymore because I was in the other bedroom "partying" all night. One night I heard something downstairs, went down to look outside, and spent the rest of the night looking out the window. I don't know who or what was out there, I just knew there was something, and I was determined to see it. When I went upstairs to shower in the morning my wife asked, "Have you been up looking out the window all night?" I said, "No." She yelled, "Liar! Go look in the mirror." I had lines embedded in my face from the blinds.

Realizing I'd been busted, I set the dope on the side and started drinking again. I'd stay up in the other bedroom drinking a fifth of booze a night. As you can imagine, if you drink a fifth of booze a night, you're eventually going to have to go to the bathroom, but I couldn't because then my wife would know I was up drinking. I spotted this plant in the corner of the room and started relieving myself there. One night when I came home from work, the plant was at the end of the driveway in the garbage. When I asked what was up with my plant, my wife told me she had to throw it out because of the stench.

My ridiculous behavior continued as I joined the "wreck-a-car-a-month" club. I stopped going to work altogether, and I began shooting at chirping birds that disturbed me when I was trying to sleep. Still, I could not see what the drugs and the booze were doing to me. I could only feel what they were doing for me, and I was trapped in a downward spiral.

I couldn't take it anymore, so I went to my firm and told them I needed a change. I offered them a two-year noncompetition contract in return for two years' pay. They said, "Done. Goodbye," and cut me a check. The money was gone within 30 days; I drank, drugged, and gambled it all away.

The hope ran out of my life. The businesses were gone, I was unemployed and unemployable, I had seemingly insurmountable debt, and my wife was filing for divorce. I was down to two homes—my car and the gas station bathroom. I was completely and absolutely alone. I had taken out a flamethrower and burned my life to the ground. The party train had hit the end of the line and derailed in a fiery crash. The pain was too great, and I could no longer kill it, so I went to a hotel room to die.

As I sat alone in that room, I began having flashbacks. I had visions of the lifeless body of a guy I jammed in a brawl, and of my wife lying in a fetal position on the bed, crying because there was no money for food or diapers. I had a vision of my beautiful little one-year-old daughter shaking and cowering in the corner, fearing that her daddy was going to go into a rage again.

I gave up and acknowledged that there was no way I could handle this by myself any more. I begged for mercy: "Please, God, I don't want to die like this, but I don't want to live like this any more, either. God, please help me."

The reply I got was interesting: "Go help yourself."

Somehow I landed on the doorstep of Cocaine Anonymous. I was a mess, completely devoid of any decent living instincts. I was 29 years old, and I had nothing. I had stopped wondering long ago who I was, but rather wondered what I was. I took stock: I'm an alcoholic, a drug addict, a compulsive gambler, and an overeater; I'm addicted to money, sex, and power. Beautiful! You name it, I had it. I could have been the poster child for "A Whole Pile of Crap Anonymous." I asked myself, "What am I doing at C.A. when my problem with cocaine is just the tip of the iceberg? What the heck do I do now?"

I did what everybody else was doing: I got myself a sponsor. I picked a guy ahead of me in sobriety who was actively sponsored and sponsoring others. I chose him because he was working the Steps, involved in the Fellowship, and knew everybody wherever we went. I picked him because he showed people how it works with his eyes and his actions, not by passive dictating. I chose him because he shared his experience in recovery, and when he shared his story, it was as though he was describing me. He had been where I was.

Choosing strong, hard-nosed, and enthusiastic sponsorship and allowing myself to be sponsored are quite simply the most important gifts I have ever given to myself. My sponsor did not try to dictate my life, but helped me survive until I could get the hope, faith and courage to make the necessary changes. He instilled in me a structure of actions and follow-through, of making commitments to others and myself. He ingrained in me enough trust in him for me to accept his judgment over my distorted opinions.

I took actions at his direction that I never would have taken otherwise, not for anyone. He set me up with a predetermined set of lifesaving habits. He taught me the one thing that I hang on to each and every day: if I continue to take the actions, I will continue to get better, and if I stop taking the actions, I will get worse, but I might not see it immediately because I have a blind spot to the unmanageability in my life.

My sponsor started me taking action. He got me to start doing what I said I was going do when I said I was going to do it. He coaxed me into being polite, and he told me I needed to smile because I was the crabbiest guy he'd ever seen. He suggested that I never say "no" to a C.A. request; I figured that should be easy because I couldn't imagine anybody asking me to do anything but leave without stealing the money. He had me get to meetings early, introduce myself to the chairperson, and ask if I could read a portion of the format. After a while, he suggested I introduce myself to the people in the Fellowship that I didn't know and always say hello to newcomers. He instilled in me the idea that we must never let a newcomer feel alone because we don't have to be alone any more, ever again.

It wasn't long before I knew people all over this Fellowship, and I was doing service work all over the place. Without knowing it, I was suddenly a part of. My whole world was changing. I learned that if I don't behave offensively, people don't respond defensively towards me. The stuff my sponsor was teaching me was working, and my life was drastically improving.

Before I got here, I thought my problem was that I drank and drugged too much. What I learned was that the drugs and the booze are but symptoms of our disease. I learned that my problem is not that I drink and I drug too much, but that I'm powerless. If the problem is that I'm powerless, quite simply, the solution has got to be to find the power—to experience the spiritual awakening necessary to recover from addiction.

My sponsor expressed the importance of sticking with the winners. We discussed how I am prone to change my personality to blend in with my background. This means that I must stick with people who are enthusiastically seeking recovery because they're moving in a positive direction; when I have no direction to go in myself, I adjust to them and keep going. If I want to stay enthusiastic in my pursuit of recovery, hanging around half-steppers will likely choke off my enthusiasm—not because they're sick, but because I am.

So I took the suggested actions and did all the service work I could handle, side by side with others who were doing their best to stay sober. My sponsor and I were attacking the Steps. We worked Steps One through Three, and I felt the power of two addicts coming together for the sole purpose of recovery. When my head told me to get high even though in my heart I wanted sobriety, I'd get with people in recovery, and I could not go back out there. I came to believe that there is power when we come together, and I found hope that there is a solution. I made a decision to work on my relationship with my Higher Power, and I learned this through the people here. I truly believe that God introduced me to Cocaine Anonymous, and the people in Cocaine Anonymous introduced me to God. In working Steps

One, Two, and Three, I also righted myself to the concept of a Higher Power.

In Steps Four through Seven, I got a handle on myself. Through working the Steps with my sponsor, I began to see the nature of my defects, the attitudes that drive my thinking and block my path to the power. These defects are what must be changed.

As I worked Steps Eight and Nine, I got right in relationship with my fellow man. Suddenly God, you, and I came together in the universe. I looked around and realized that the Promises were showing up in my life, and the obsession to drink and drug was gone.

We went on to Step Ten, and I started working Steps Four through Nine daily. Through this process, I started developing an intuition, a sixth sense about living. My perception is that we are spiritual creatures, born into this world out of love and sent out on this earth to love. I view the Steps as a design for spiritual creatures having a human experience.

How do I keep this going? How do I keep the power? Prayer and meditation. I pray and ask God for direction, and I meditate to hear the answers. When I listen in silence, I hear; and it is in silence that God and I come face to face.

The Steps didn't care how sincere I was. I didn't work these Steps because I cared about you; I did this stuff because my sponsor told me this was the only way out. I thought I didn't care about you, but then God threw in a wild card, and I discovered that I did. When I love and care about you, it feels like you love and care about me—and that's all I ever wanted. Right here in the program of Cocaine Anonymous I found everything I ever needed to heal those empty holes in my soul, and I came to believe in a God that will never let me down.

Through working the Twelve Steps, I came face to face with my Higher Power, the spirit that moves through the universe and is transmitted by the people in the Fellowship. To tap into the power, I must get with the people. Having had a spiritual awakening as the result of these Steps, I feel the power, and now that I've found the power, I have to transmit the power.

So I'm here with my sponsees and other enthusiastic sober folks, continuing to take the actions, work with others, and carry the message of hope, faith and courage. We're smiling and laughing, going to meetings, studying the literature, working the Steps, screwing things up, making them right, doing H&I service work, making new friends, being parents and partners, and having the time of our spiritually imperfect lives.

Why do I keep taking these actions after all these years? Not because I'm a wonderful guy, or some crazed recovery zealot. I keep taking these actions simply because I love my life today, and the actions I've been taking since the day I walked in here have yet to fail me. The buzz of life keeps getting bigger and bigger, and the reward keeps getting better and better.

If you're new to recovery, welcome to the party! I want you to know I've been where you've been, I've thought the way you thought, I've felt the way you felt, and I've acted the way you acted. You see, I walked in here a broken-down shell of a man. I rebuilt my life based on the Twelve-Step recovery program of Cocaine Anonymous. Because I jumped into this program with both feet and without reservation, I'm here to tell you that I've got a great life. I am living the dream.

God has touched me with many gifts: to feel loved and cared for, to feel a part of, and to feel comfortable enough in my own skin to not pick up a drink or a drug today. All anybody has ever asked of me in return is that I pass it on. God has blessed me with the gift of sobriety; may He bless you, too!

6

NORMAL ON THE OUTSIDE

Cocaine Anonymous taught her it was an inside job.

I was sitting on a plane, taking a transatlantic flight back to the city where I was born, and wondering to myself, "What happened? How had this happened to me? When did I stop using drugs and they start using me? How had I become this person that I could no longer recognize?"

This was not a trip I wanted to make. I was returning with no money, no job, no home to go to, friendless and just wanting to go to a corner and curl up and die. Although at the time I was not aware of the names for the feelings I was experiencing, I later found out that they were despair, hopelessness, and shame; I felt a complete failure, empty and lonely.

A few years back I had been living in a midtown apartment in the biggest city in the world, making tons of money, having all the stuff that made me think and feel good enough, and I kidded myself that I had it made. In truth, my life even then was a sham, but I thought I had control. I was snorting lots of cocaine and taking other combinations of mind-altering substances to go up or down, or this way or that, zigzagging; but I kept up appearances.

Growing up in the northwest suburbs of London, I knew from the earliest age what it was that a good girl "should" do and how to keep up appearances. There was always an assumption that I would meet a man, get married, and have children. That was the message, and that was the experience of the families around me, and that's what did happen to my sister, cousins, and school friends. In my home we were adept at keeping up appearances, and so long as we dressed well, smiled, and went on the right holidays, everything was fine. Of course, inside our home things were far from all right. My father was a raging, compulsive gambler, and I learnt to mask my feelings from the earliest age. I thought this was normal. Living with that addiction meant constant uncertainty—all-or-nothing behaviour around me and lots of denial. My mother adapted to my father's moods and protected us from most of the emotional onslaught. We never spoke about this; we just went shopping, and I was very protected by the rest of my family.

I had many friends, from several different groups, and I was good at becoming who you wanted me to be. I quickly developed different behaviours, depending on who I was with or where I was going. Growing up in the 1960s, I embraced the concept of sex, drugs, rock-and-roll, and my heroes were the rock bands and fashion icons that were so groundbreaking at the time. I discovered pot and pills, and in the early years of my addiction loved the feeling they gave me. It was quite socially acceptable to get high, and I scorned those who tried to warn me of the dangers of using drugs.

Fast-forward a few years: my survival skills were razor sharp at the grand age of 16. I was living in the centre of town and thinking of myself as all grown up. My mother had died the year before after a long illness, and the whole family fell to pieces. I was coping and had left school, left my family, left the suburbs, and all the restrictions of authority. In all truth I just didn't care about much. I had already adopted my motto of "live fast, party hard, and die young"... and the path ahead was set.

In retrospect, I see that I went through the classic progression of addiction. The only drug that was taboo for me was heroin. I had a friend who died of an overdose when I was 13, and the message I got was clear: don't mess with that, but everything else was fair play.

During the next 20 years, although I moved to different cities and countries, backward and forward, I kept taking the problem, me, with me. Cocaine had taken a grip, and my addiction was the driving force behind my choices and decisions. I compared myself with those around me and could always find another person who appeared worse off. This enabled me to believe things were still okay, that I had control. When I moved from the straw to the pipe, I knew inside that now I had a problem. But my solution was to blame it on my man or other people, and it was always someone else's fault that I had messed up yet again.

The last years of my using were like living in the twilight zone, being one of the living dead. Those around me were like-minded, so I normalized the abnormal. Spending days without sleep was standard; so were buying, selling, and using. Cocaine was what my life centred around, and it came before everything. I acquired a husband and stepdaughters who were also users, and I blamed them for the chaos in my life. I tried to stop; a detox, a holiday, getting rid of all the paraphernalia—nothing worked. I exchanged my husband for my dealer, and things got worse. Eventually I had a moment of clarity and saw that the problem was me. With all the usual drama, I packed my bags and got on that plane, broken and hopeless.

I was Twelve-Stepped by a friend of my family. I have no idea why I got it without a struggle. It was nearing winter in 1992 when my Higher Power led me into a treatment centre in the English countryside. I had no idea of what to expect, only my fantasies that I was entering a health spa where I would get personal attention, beauty treatments, therapy, etc., for the next six weeks. I brought with me magazines, a stash of pain killers and a feeling of disillusionment and desperation. I had no concept of total abstinence and did not know that I was suffering from a chronic and killer disease. My experience over the next six weeks was profound. I was blessed with the ability to listen and learn that I was suffering from the disease of addiction and that there was a solution through the Twelve Steps. I found the Fellowship of Cocaine Anonymous by accident, and I knew immediately that I had found my spiritual home—identification, laughter, and a place to belong, an instant family.

I was encouraged to be honest, open-minded, and willing. I applied myself to Step work with the same resolve and tenacity that I had applied to my using. I desired recovery, and all around me I saw that those who had what I wanted were doing certain things: prayer, meetings, Step work, service, and putting their recovery above and beyond everything else. So I tried to the best of my ability to do the same. The first year certainly had its challenges, being homeless, jobless, and still very wrecked from the damage from my past. It was also the most exciting time, when I rediscovered how to laugh, to feel emotion, to share my shame and be okay, to be part of the early days of Cocaine Anonymous in my area.

I kept doing the next right thing one day at a time, and I found the desire to use had vanished. I continued to work the Steps with a sponsor and found in time that I was able to pass the message on to sponsees. I went back to education and attained a degree in law, then I changed my mind and decided I wanted a different career. Through the Eighth and Ninth Steps, I repaired many old relationships and became the sister I had never been, the aunt I had hoped to be, a good friend to my friends, and in time there was substance and love in my relationships with those about me.

Starting with my first commitment as tea/coffee person, I have always been very involved in service to the Fellowship of Cocaine Anonymous. I got to know everyone and found by getting there early and staying late, it was easy to feel "part of." Throughout the years of my recovery, I have continued to be blessed by being able to be of service. This has brought great spiritual rewards and has allowed me to learn and grow as a human being. I thank God that I remain teachable and that my journey has brought many wonderful people and teachers into my life. Recently I have been able to be witness to and help support our Fellowship as it grows in new countries and to see again that no matter where we are, no matter which language, culture or country, the Twelve-Step programme of Cocaine Anonymous works. This has truly been fabulous and a gift to be part of.

Along the road there have been pain and difficulties. My father died a few years ago; I have seen my sister in a coma in intensive care; my partner lost his business and with that all our material and financial security. At those times I continued to do what I was shown: trust God, share honestly, and help others. I know, with certainty in my heart, that the programme of Cocaine Anonymous works, no matter what life throws at me—the good times, the bad times, all times.

Throughout this journey I have seen miracles. I have seen the desire and obsession to use removed not only in my life but also in the lives of countless others. I have witnessed hopelessness turn to hope and on to joy in the lives of so many of those around me. I know this gift is precious, and keeping it relies on my being of service and continuing to work the Twelfth Step on a daily basis. The wonderful thing is that for me today, I couldn't think of a better way to live, and I thank God, Cocaine Anonymous, and the wonderful members of our Fellowship—those I know, those I hope to know, and those who came before me—for the opportunity to live life, have a life and value that life.

7

GETTING UNSTUCK

One addict's journey from emergency rooms to the rooms of recovery.

I was raised in the projects. My house was "the house." Tricks got turned in my bedroom, and stolen items were fenced in my house. All types of illegal activity went on in my home, and this is what I was raised up seeing.

My mother was the neighborhood alcoholic, drug addict, whatever, and she was the fall-down type of drunk. She would do things like urinate in the middle of the sidewalk in broad daylight, and I would have to go to school and hear about how my mother performed. I was embarrassed, and I was ridiculed.

She also wasn't able to help me keep up with fads like designer clothing. My mother would get me clothes from churches and shelters and things like that. Sometimes there would be designer clothing in the bag, but it wouldn't always be my size. So what I would do was take some scissors and cut the little insignia out, and I would sew it or glue it onto a regular T-shirt. If you know anything about most designer logos, that's not a patch, that's actual stitching in the shirt. So I would try to cut with precision, and I would sew it or glue it onto another shirt, and I would go to school like I had the real thing. And I guess my logo must have been crooked, and they'd be like, "Man, let me see the inside of that shirt." And I'd be, like, "Man, I gotta go to class!"

Also, when I was growing up, I was so badly cross-eyed that it was like my eyes sat on the bridge of my nose. That was real rough on me because I would be talking to someone, and I'd be like, "Hey, you want to go to the store?" and he would turn and look to see who I was talking to. I thought I was looking at him eye to eye, but I guess not.

I remember this girl in my school. I liked her, and I told her I wanted her to be my girl. She said, "You know, you're cute and everything, but I can't talk to you because you're cross-eyed." If she didn't like the way I dressed, I could have got some more clothes. If she didn't like my hair, I could have got some waves or something. She picked the one thing about me that I had absolutely no control over, and I was devastated. I knew I had no chance at all with this girl because I couldn't fix my eyes.

I got beat up a lot in my neighborhood. I didn't get beat up because I was scared to fight, I got beat up because I was scared to win. In my neighborhood, if you get in a fight and you win, you gotta fight the next day. Then if you win the next day, you have to fight the next day after that. And if you win too many times, you gotta fight their big brother or their crazy cousin. I figure, beat me up today, and get all the rest of that fightin' out of the way right now! Then I got this bright idea. I decide to start hanging with the guys that beat me up, and maybe we'll just beat other people up.

So I'm hanging out with these guys, they got some marijuana, they got some beer, and we're getting high. I don't know what alcohol or drugs did for anybody else, but when I smoked that weed and I drank that beer, I looked in the mirror and said, "Man, this is alright!" I felt stronger and more confident, and it didn't matter what my mother was or wasn't doing. My clothes were adequate. My eyes were straight. Alcohol did something for me that I couldn't do for myself. So at 11 or 12 years old, I made up my mind, "I have to stay high. If I do not stay high, I'm going to feel the way that I felt before, and I can't have that."

I was about 14 years old, and my mother had different men in and out of the house, and there was all the stuff I was doing, and she told me to leave if I couldn't follow the rules of her house. So I left. I experienced homelessness. I slept in "condemned-o-miniums" and abandoned cars, and I was okay with it because after I woke up out of that abandoned building, I got to be grown up. I started hanging out with these guys that were older than me. They smoked weed all day, so I smoked weed all day. They drank all day, so I drank all day. One day we were all sitting in the hallway, and they pulled out all of this stuff, like some type of chemistry experiment. They broke out this light-bulb type of instrument, and they had some alcohol and scissors and cotton balls and hangers, and I'm wondering, "What the hell are they doing?"

So one guy lit the scissors, and he put it on the light bulb, and his eyes got big, and he got real jittery. And then another guy did the same thing and got so jittery and shaky he couldn't talk. Then another guy hit it, and he got jittery and shaky and couldn't talk. They said, "You want to hit this?" I said, "Yeah!" They told me, "Put it in your mouth, and pull it like a cigarette." I did. My eyes didn't get big, and I didn't get jittery, and I didn't go through the changes they went through. I said to myself, "Whatever that is, I won't be messing with that, it's a waste of time." What I know today is they handed me an empty pipe. But that's when I first started smokin' crack cocaine.

By the time I was 16, I was fully addicted. I had people two and three times my age looking at me saying, "Damn, at least I'm not that bad." I did just about anything and everything to get high. The things that I did not do, I would have done them if somebody had approached me right on one of them nights when I was geeking for real. I would have been sayin', "You ain't gonna tell nobody, is you?" Because I'd have done anything for one more. That's all my life consisted of—one more. After I got one more, all I wanted was one more. And that's what my life was.

I started running customers for this guy, and these people pulled up and they wanted something. It was the amount of money that I needed, so I hooked them up. I'm ready to get paid, but because I'm greedy, I'm telling the people at the car, "Y'all going to hook me up, too—right?" So they hook me up, and I run around the corner to catch the guy, and when I run around the corner, this other guy was robbing him. And I said, "Don't rob him, man! He's cool. If you're going to get anybody, don't get him!" The bottom line was the guy was about to rob him and take the dope, and I didn't want him to take the dope. I should have been saying, "Please don't take the dope!"

After he got finished being robbed I said to him, "Man, you okay? That's messed up!" He said, "Yeah, I'm okay, but you won't be because I know you set me up." I honestly had nothing to do with it, but I went and hid in someone's house because these guys were known killers. The least thing they would do to you is shoot you. If they shot you, you was getting off easy. So I'm hiding under the bed, and these eight guys come in and snatch me. All of them had different kinds of guns, and one had a pit bull. They commenced to kick me, beat me, stomp me, pistol-whip me, and then they let the pit bull loose on me. He started biting and shaking my arms. He locked onto my chin and was shaking my face. He locked onto my ear and ripped it in half. He locked onto the back of my neck and bit a hole in it. I remember screaming, but I wasn't screaming from pain, I was screaming from fear. I thought this was just a warm-up for the bullet. But they pulled the dog off of me, kicked and beat me some more, and then they left.

Now when I got up I looked in the mirror and I was very badly bruised and beaten. My ear was hanging off my head. The back of my neck was bleeding. There were a whole bunch of teeth marks in my arms. Then I put my hands in my pockets and felt the $4 that the people had given me for hooking them up. I know I'm messed up and I need to go to the hospital, but I'm thinking I'll get me a $4 piece before I go.

I looked in the mirror and as torn up as I was, I knew that that was worth a piece by itself! I knew that somebody would feel sorry for me as bad a shape as I was in. I went around knocking on people's doors, and they opened the door, like, "Man! What the hell happened to you?" I said, "I was selling a little something, and some guys robbed me." They said, "Well, go to the hospital!" I said, "I am, right after I get me a $4 piece! Can you hook me up?"

I remember another time I went down to the emergency room after getting stabbed with an ice pick during a deal that went bad, and the nurses and doctors were checking me out, giving me a tetanus shot, and looking at my wounds. I told them, "Can you all just leave for a minute? I just need to be alone, get my head together." I lay on the emergency bed, smokin' bloody rocks out of an antenna with some matches. And I didn't think I had a problem!

Another time this guy gave me some rocks to sell for him, and I'm out there all night. I've only got one problem with selling dope, personally: I had to taste it first, you know. And once I taste it, I get stuck. You know, you ask me how it is, and I won't be there to tell you.

So the guy gave me ten $20 rocks, and I go in the hallway and taste one, and I get stuck. I can't talk, and I can't move so I'm just sitting there. I'm looking at the dope, and I chip off another piece because the only way for me to get unstuck is to take another hit. (It's kind of baffling how I can't move or talk when I get stuck, but I can grab a rock and a lighter.) I'm sitting there with ten $20s, and I'm chipping off of them, and I'm smoking. I've got ten $20s, then I've got five $20s, then I've got four $10s, then I've got eight $2.76 pieces. I think, "Ain't nobody going to buy this. I'm smokin' it."

Now this guy's going to crack my head, right? So I say, "Man, I think I need some treatment." I first came to the rooms of recovery in 1994, but not because I wanted some help. I went to treatment for the same reason a lot of people go to treatment—to get some rest.

In treatment, they told me, "You know, you need to go to meetings." I went to a meeting, and this guy was standing behind the podium, and he said, "I lost my wife because of drinking. I lost my job because of drinking. I wrecked my car because of drinking. My kids don't love me because of drinking." And I'm sitting in the back of the room thinking, "Man, this is depressing! They want me to come here and listen to that, to help me?" I wanted to find the dude when he came out of the meeting and get him a wine, that's how depressed I was sitting in the back of the room. I wasn't identifying.

They told me to read the "Big Book," and I said, "Man, ain't no way in the world a book written by two middle-class white men in the 1930s is gonna help a brother from the gutter in the 1990s."

They told me to get a sponsor. I said, "I don't want to put nobody in my business."

The inevitable happened: I got drunk, and I got high. A lot of people in the Fellowship will tell you, "He got high because he wanted to get high," or, "She got high because she wanted to get high," but I know now that I have no mental defense against the first drink. If I'm not building a working relationship with God, I'm going to do what comes naturally, and that's get high.

I went back out there, but even though I wasn't listening, I'd heard some things in the meetings. "You do not have to continue to live like this." I'm hearing these voices: "It's not the last one, it's the first one." I'm smokin' and I'm trying to concentrate and I'm already hearing voices anyway, and then I'm hearing this recovery stuff, so I'm going crazy trying to get high.

I came back in here and I questioned everything. They said, "Read the book." I said, "Why?" They said, "Work the Steps." I said, "Why?" They said, "Get a sponsor." I said, "Why?" I never asked the corner store owner, "Why is your roses wild?" I never said, "Hey, man, we're from Colombia. Who cut this?" I wasn't interested in the minor details. You told me what a drug would do to me and I took it, but I come into recovery and I want to dictate to people how they should help me. They'd tell me what to do, and I'd say, "Well, I'll do this and this, but I ain't gonna do that and that," but if I don't know anything about staying sober, I'm going to pick the wrong thing, and my ass is going to be drunk.

It's important that I do what's being told to me to do and leave the results up to God. I'm going to learn by doing, not by knowing. I don't have to know how God works in order for Him to work in my life. I've just got to believe in Him. That's what happened for me.

I came back into the program, and I got with some individuals who were practicing this program. I read about how this disease has three parts: a physical allergy, a mental obsession, and a spiritual malady. I learned about the physical allergy and the phenomenon of craving, and how my alcoholic/addict body is as abnormal as my mind.

I relate. If I'm allergic to strawberries and I eat a strawberry, it's going to make me break out. But I'm smart. I figure that maybe if I mix some ice cream and milk in a blender with some strawberries, the milk and ice cream will break down the potency of the strawberries, and it won't make me break out. But it does. So I'm *real* smart. I'm going to wait five years, change my name, move to a fine neighborhood, buy a luxury car, get married, and then I'll eat a strawberry. Guess what's going to happen? It's still going to make me break out.

No matter where I live, who I date, how much money I make, or where I get high, that stuff is going to do exactly what it did to me the last time I used it. Period. I had to take an honest look at my life. I discovered that it don't matter how or where I use. If I put a little piece on, use a little bit of chore, smoke it longways instead of lengthways, Park Avenue, park bench, it don't matter! No matter how much weight I gain, where I live, where I move, or who I know, my insides will never change. Dope and alcohol is going to do to me exactly what it did to me the last time I used it. Period. And that was important for me to understand.

The physical allergy hits me in many different forms. One that sticks out the most for me is the high before the high. I ain't even started gettin' high yet, and I'm sweating, I'm jittery, I'm trippin', but I ain't smoked nothin'! Just the thought of getting high got my body going through changes.

The other part is that once I put drugs or alcohol in me, I can't determine when it's going to end. My disease takes everything that I have, and then it demands more. After I'm out of all of my money, after I've lied and stolen and cheated everybody I can cheat, I sit alone in my house and come up with things like, "You're rarely ever in the living room man, sell that couch!" Or, "What do you need with two TVs, you're always in one room. Sell that!" And then I sell it.

You know, a lot of people say, "Drugs robbed me of this," or "Alcohol robbed me of that." Well, a running stem ain't never jumped in my mouth and lit itself. This mind tells these hands to get into these pockets and buy that stuff. So it all starts with this mind. I can't blame anything or anybody for the reason I am who and what I am.

I'll give an example of the mental obsession. I get some money, and I go over to these people's house, and when I get there I'm the man. They pat me on my back, they co-sign everything I say, "Yeah, son, yeah!" They go to the store for me. They're willing to do things for me. But I get down to the last of my dope, and they start yawning. Now it's time for the dethroning process because my dope's gone. So I get up, I leave. I say, "Screw them! They ain't ever gotta worry about me coming back over there!" And I mean that. That day. I mean that that week. I even mean that on payday. But pay moment, when that money hits my hands ... you know what happens. I will repeat this over and over again, and unless I experience a spiritual awakening as the result of working the Steps, there's very little hope for my recovery.

I was obsessed. Even my solutions involved me getting high. I had a great idea—y'all probably never thought of this. Put $300 in my sock and $20 in my pocket! That's actually a good idea, except after I take a hit, I know where I hid the money at. And my mind makes a quick plan in getting that sock, man. I'm obsessed. At the end I said that I didn't want to do this no more, but I was making a firm resolution with an obsessed mind. My mind thinks about nothing but getting high, so how can I use my sick mind to heal itself?

Another part of my disease is that I have soul sickness. I'll do anything to get high—*anything*. I'd steal from my grandmother. If somebody said, "Man, how could you steal from your grandmother?" I'd say, "Man, that wasn't my grandmother. That was a lick!" Now after I sober up, I say, "Damn, man, why do I steal from my grandma?"

When I look at my life honestly, I'm a liar, a thief, a con, a manipulator, selfish, self-centered, dishonest, self-seeking, frightened, egotistical; I have drug problems, I drink—I've got, like 15 major issues! You think if I quit smoking dope I'll be running around here happy? I'm going to be miserable because I've got all these issues, and I can't even drink.

The Twelve Steps are designed to help me deal with those issues. That's their purpose. I get better by working the Twelve Steps. If I don't want to change and if I don't want to get better, then I need to leave the Steps alone. The strange thing about the Twelve Steps is that they work even if I don't work them. They just won't work for me.

I suffered from terminal uniqueness when I got here because I was 21 years old when I got sober, but I'd had an eight-year run just like a lot of people in recovery. When I got here, I was unwilling. I didn't want to listen. I didn't want to follow instructions, but it's vital that I listen to somebody. I cannot allow my thinking to run my life. I have to get with some older members of this program and allow them to help me, without reservation. I have to do what's in front of me to do and leave the results up to God.

I'm a proud member of Cocaine Anonymous. The reason why I love Cocaine Anonymous so much is because I get to tell the whole truth here. Some places you go they don't want you to talk about dope. They want you to talk about "side dishes" and other stuff. I didn't do no damn "side dishes." I smoked dope out of a pipe and with some chore. I came to Cocaine Anonymous so I could free myself, and I could tell people just like me about me, and they would understand me.

I'm really not "all that." If I said anything in my story to help anybody, give credit to God and the Twelve Steps of Cocaine Anonymous.

8

BIRTHMARK

A stray bullet was the beginning of a new life.

I grew up in a single-parent household in which discipline and hard work were emphasized. My mother wanted the best for me and my sister, and she worked hard to provide a pleasant atmosphere in which to live. We had a roof over our heads, food to eat, and nice clothes to wear. We couldn't always participate in some school activities because of money, but my mother did her best. After some time in recovery, I realize how good I had it as a kid, but as a child I could only see the negative in my life. Because of my mother's work schedule and the fact that she grew up in a home where emotions were not displayed or honored, I felt lonely most of the time. When I tried to express how I felt to my mother or anyone else in my family, I was judged ungrateful and strange.

As a result, I tended to isolate as a child and escaped into the wonderful world of books. When I read, I could become anyone I wanted to be and escape from my reality. I also discovered food. As a child I loved to curl up with a book and some sweet treat and pretend to be someone else living a different life. Little did I know that this type of behavior would lay the foundation for my life of fantasizing.

The one place where my light blazed brightly was in school. I basked in my mother's admiration when she showed others my grade cards and school awards. I loved the attention and scaled higher and higher heights of academia to ensure that I would always have her love. I confused attention with love; I thought if you paid attention to me then you must surely love me.

I carried my coping skills to school, and high school was a world like no other. The classes were more challenging, and I, who had always easily made good grades, became an average student. I was chunky (a consequence of all that reading and eating), which did not help my social ambitions at all. I didn't fit into any of the different cliques. I didn't come from a family with money, so I couldn't hang out in the rich crowd; I had become an average student, so hanging out with the geeks was not an option.

In my junior year of high school, I became pregnant. This increased the distance between my mother and myself, since I was now a disgrace to her. I had my daughter and continued with school, but I felt alone again, and this time the books and food did not fill the void.

I carried this empty, lonely feeling around with me until one day I noticed another type of crowd on the school bus. They hung out in the back, and they always seemed real cool. Everybody seemed to admire them, and they were invited to the best parties at school. I noticed a brown paper bag was passed among them some days, and on others the smell of marijuana would drift to the front of the bus. I thought to myself that they were having fun and that maybe I should see what was up with them.

Each day I sat a row closer to the back of the bus, until one day there I was in the back of bus with the cool crowd. A joint was coming my way, and I couldn't look uncool since appearances were very important to me. I took a drag off of it and pounded my chest. I felt nothing from the joint, but what I did feel was the immediate acceptance by the cool crowd. It felt wonderful. I had their attention and acceptance. I had arrived! I associated with this group until I graduated from high school.

After I graduated from high school, I attended college for one year. I was enrolled to be a nurse. My motives for going to nursing school were not so that I could help sick people but so that I could make money in a career that would always be in demand. I shudder to think of the treatment some of my patients would have experienced. However, one of my character defects was impatience, and nursing school was going to take four years. I quit school and started going from job to job. I always blamed the job for not being the "right" job. I never took a look at myself to see what part I played.

My drug use now included alcohol, marijuana, and ecstasy. I was a neglectful mother and partied every weekend. I reasoned that if you had a life like mine, you would get high, too. One summer my marijuana and ecstasy connections dried up. I tried to drink my restlessness away, but the alcohol did not do the job for me. I was not used to being in my own skin without some sort of mind-altering substance. I was sitting around brainstorming one night with a girlfriend of mine, thinking, "What can I get high on?" I came up with the idea of trying crack, and my swift downward slide began. With the first hit I knew I was in trouble because the words I said were, "I have found heaven."

I maintained a semblance of normality for a time, but it was becoming more and more apparent that something was not right in my life. I started out only using on weekends, but soon every day became a weekend. I would rationalize and say, "Oh, I am just going to buy a $20 rock," and twenty $20s later I would beat my chest and say, "How did I get here again?" I started missing work and was late to pick up my daughter from school, if I showed up at all. I had always been promiscuous, but with crack cocaine in my life, I sank lower and lower in my dealings with men. Eventually I sent my daughter to live in another city with my mother. This allowed me to start partying full force. I lived to use, and even though I no longer enjoyed the high or the people, I couldn't stop. I was miserable.

One Friday as I was driving to get my beer and my first $20, there was a gunfight going down on the street I was traveling. I saw the guys shoot at each other, and my smoking companion who was with me suggested that maybe we should turn around. I told him, "No, they are shooting at each other, and they are not going to shoot at us."

Then a bullet came through the windshield. First I felt pressure on my forehead, then it was like someone had turned on a faucet. I felt a warm sensation coming down my face. I realized that it was blood, flowing heavily, and I couldn't see the road. My smoking buddy said, "Maybe you should pull over," but I said, "No, I can see." He finally convinced me to stop. The paramedics were called, and I was rushed to the hospital, where I had surgery to remove the broken glass from my forehead. Amazingly, the bullet had only grazed my forehead, and I still have the scar to this day. I call it my birthmark because it marked the beginning of my new life. From that point on, I knew that I had a serious problem.

I had been through an outpatient treatment program before, and I called one of the counselors I had befriended. She recommended C.A. I had never heard of C.A., but at that point I was willing to try anything. I knew that if I continued to get high, I was going to die. The next time, the bullet might not miss.

I started attending C.A. meetings, and I was willing to do anything. When I first heard *Who is a Cocaine Addict?* read, I was immediately hooked—just like the first time I tried crack. I fell in love with C.A. and felt at home immediately. I heard people share stories like mine, and since they had recovered, I got busy right away!

They told me to make coffee, and I said, "How many pots?"

They said, "Chair a meeting!" Well, I was scared, but I was more scared not to, so I did it anyway.

They said, "Get a sponsor!" I found a male sponsor. Today I do not personally recommend that if you are a woman, but at that time it worked for me.

They said, "Get involved in service!" and so I did.

Most importantly, they said, "Work the Steps," and I started the wonderful, beautiful process of uncovering, discovering, and recovering.

Through writing my Fourth Step and then sharing it in my Fifth, I came to realize that my mother had done the very best she could with what was given her and that my tendency to concentrate on the negative did not help matters. We now have a solid relationship, and today I have gratitude for her efforts to raise us right. I have also found a way to deal with my emotions positively by praying, inventorying, and sharing them with my sponsor and others in my support network.

My daughter moved back in with me, and I soberly brought her up through those hair-raising teen years. She will be graduating from college next year. I have been at my present job for over six years with many promotions. That is a miracle for an addict like me. I moved some years ago to a place where there were no C.A. meetings, so I started one. Cocaine Anonymous is booming, and it is a joy to see the light come on in other people's eyes. This is an experience you really must not miss. I have over nine years clean, and that is another miracle. Thank you, HP, for blessing me with C.A.

9

A LIFE WORTH LIVING

By doing the best he could each day of his recovery and leaving the results up to God, he experienced a life beyond his wildest expectations.

When I first came into the rooms of Cocaine Anonymous, I heard someone identify as a "grateful" addict/alcoholic. For the life of me I couldn't figure out how anyone could be grateful to be an addict and an alcoholic. I thought perhaps this person was simply grateful not to be drinking and using anymore. After the meeting, I approached the grateful individual, and he confirmed that he was actually grateful to be an addict/alcoholic.

"Because if I wasn't a drug addict and an alcoholic," he shared with me, "whose life depended on working all 12 of those Steps, I never would have done it." Further, he explained, by working the Twelve Steps of Cocaine Anonymous, he had not just been given his life back, but had been given a life worth living.

When I got here, I had a problem with living. From the time I was a child I had always wanted to be someone else, somewhere else, doing something else. Drugs and alcohol allowed me to escape temporarily. In my heart of hearts, I felt that I could never be the person I wanted to be, so I spent many years trying to escape life through drugs and alcohol, and that temporary fix was all I had. Every time I quit drinking and using, I would look around at life and say to myself, "Yep, life sucks. That's why I drink and use. I can't stand this."

Over time, my tolerance became greater, my need for more drugs increased, and the ability to escape into the unreality of a euphoric fantasy world dissipated. In the end I found myself locked inside my house with the curtains drawn and pinned closed, hitting a freebase pipe and wondering to myself, "Is that a crack in the curtain?"

Completely paranoid at 3 a.m., I believed that someone on the outside might see the flame of my torch and come inside. If they were the police, they would arrest me. If they were burglars, they would rob me and take my last precious stash. My best solution was to go into the closet to use. I figured that maybe "they" wouldn't be able to see into the closet. Utter insanity.

At first drugs and alcohol were my solution, then they became my problem. When they turned on me I had nothing left, nowhere to go. I had a miserable existence. When I scored, I would use until it was all gone, and then I would pass out and start the whole process over again. I had lost my home, my family, my job, my car, my wife, and most precious of all to me, my three-year-old son and five-year-old daughter. When I was thrown out of the house and served with divorce papers, the look of disgust and hatred in their eyes tore my insides out. I couldn't blame them, however, because I hated myself.

I didn't know why I was doing what I was doing. I felt there must be something drastically wrong with me, that I must be a completely bad and evil person to do what I was doing. I hadn't wanted to be the unreliable, unfaithful husband. I didn't like the overwhelming obsession and desire that caused me to make a right turn to my dealer's house on the way to work instead of taking a left and going to the office, or to leave work with the intent of going home, only to stop by my dealer's before coming home many hours later, loaded to the gills. I didn't want to arrive hours late for appointments with my children or not show up at all.

At the end of my drinking and using, people were telling me to go away, to keep away, and that if I came back they would call the police and have me taken away. Then I found C.A., where I was told to keep coming back. The love and tolerance I experienced in these rooms was something that I had always wanted in the deepest, most recessed parts of my lonely core.

Finally I went into a hospital for treatment and called my soon-to-be-ex-wife. She had told me that if I would just admit that I had a problem, everything would be all right. I admitted it then, but when I heard her voice on the other end of the phone, it wasn't all right. She said, "That's it. You're not going to see those kids anymore." That broke my heart. It seemed drastically unfair.

Thank God for sponsors. I called mine and told him what she had said to me. His only response was, "Good. Now you have nothing to stand in the way of working the Steps." That puzzled me, but I accepted my powerlessness and started to work. I worked the Steps. I wrote. I went to meetings. I thought about the program and the Steps.

In the beginning, my sponsor asked me if I could go one day without drinking and using. I didn't think I could do that. He asked me if could go one hour. I still didn't think so. He asked me if I could go 10 minutes. I told him that I thought I could go 10 minutes. He told me that was a start. I began working this program 10 minutes at a time. He further told me that during those 10 minutes, I shouldn't call my dealer to see if he'd be home in 20 minutes.

My sponsor also told me I had to get out of the results business, that all I had to do was take the Steps and leave the rest to God. This was difficult for me because I really didn't believe in God. I knew my sponsor did. When he asked me if I believed, I didn't want to say no, so I told him the next best thing. I told him I believed in God, but God didn't like me very much; after all, look how He had screwed up my life. My sponsor said, "That's a start." We went on to the next step.

We discussed being open-minded. I told him I could not forgive the man who had murdered my father. He asked me if I was willing to forgive him; I said no. He asked me if I was willing to become willing. I thought about this for a while and decided that I could do that, but I wasn't willing to commit to it on any particular date. He said that was enough.

One of my greatest fears was that I couldn't make it in recovery. When I told my sponsor this, he told me that I had a better chance to make it if I got into service. I didn't understand how making coffee at a meeting, putting away chairs, and greeting people at the door could affect my horrible obsession to drink and use, but I had nothing to lose. I did it, and it worked.

As I got more involved, I started going to the H&I meeting of C.A. and soon had my own panels where I could go once a month into hospitals and institutions and share my story with other people. One of the things I liked best of all is that it was like having a secret weapon in my pocket. I can't tell you how many times I went to a participation meeting and heard someone share something really great, and I got to go up to them after the meeting and invite them to join me on the H&I panel. I got to build my own sobriety by working with people whose sobriety I liked, whose happiness rang through in their voices and shone in their eyes. I took them on panels, and I captured 15 to 20 minutes of their stories a couple of times a month. These people contributed directly to my sobriety. I would listen to what they said, what had happened to them, and what they did to obtain the amazing sobriety and newfound serenity that I so much craved and desired. H&I carried the message to me while I was of service.

In C.A., I was given help and direction. I was told that I could use my intellect to think about the importance of each Step. I was told to look around the rooms and find all the sober people who were working the Steps, and then stick with the winners. In going to the business meetings, doing H&I panels, and being of service, I had unconsciously surrounded myself with winners, people who were serious about the program and who were actively involved in working the Steps. I watched and emulated these people who had the sobriety that I wanted. I got sober and grew with these people.

I'm grateful to C.A. and the chances it has afforded me to be of service. I was told by my sponsor that once I get it, I have to give it away to keep it, and for me the Twelfth Step is instrumental in this. The Third Step is key to the program. When I turn my life and will over the care of God, I can't help but think that what God wants us to do is help other people. We are all God's children, and when I am into Twelfth-Step work or being of service, I am within the will of God, and I am protected, nurtured, cherished, and loved, and I have a supreme sense of euphoric serenity.

The Steps worked for me big time. I got back the love of my two children, who now give me cards on Father's Day and birthdays telling me how much I mean to them and how proud they are of me. I feel what they are really saying is how proud and grateful they are to this program and the Twelve Steps because everything I have today, everything I have achieved, is a direct result of my working the Twelve Steps of C.A. and being sober.

It happened a little bit at a time, one day at a time. When I did the best that I could to focus on today, the tomorrows I experienced surpassed even my wildest expectations. Today I have more friends than I would have ever thought possible. Today I am the type of person that I always wanted to be but never felt I could be.

I have received so many gifts: the life I always dreamed of but never felt worthy of having, a new way to look at problems, tools to search out my character defects. I have learned, as a tenet of this program, that any time I am disturbed, upset, or afraid of anything, it is because of one of my character defects. By searching them out, I may then ask God to remove them that I may be restored to sanity and peace.

Today, when I have a problem, I don't have to run and hide in a bottle. It's all about the solution for me today, about immediately looking for that which I can change—what isn't right with me, even if it's only my acceptance of the problem. I know that when I can't figure out what my character defect is, I can call my sponsor, and he will help me work it out. For the first year of my sobriety, I called him almost every day.

I am so deeply indebted to my sponsor. There was always something going on with me, and he continued to help and love me. I will love him forever and will never ever forget him or his wife. What he gave me, as he told me many times, was only what was given to him.

I remember calling him up sometime towards the end of my first year of sobriety. This time, it wasn't to complain; this time I had seen the wonderful pink cloud. I was in a state of euphoria. I told him how wonderful everything was and that my life had never been so good. He said, "Don't worry, it will get better." I told him, "No, no, no, you're not listening to me. You don't understand. I'm telling you that my life has never been this good." He said, "No. One more time, you're not listening to me. I'm telling you that if you keep doing what you're doing, your life will keep getting better."

I remained open-minded even though I couldn't imagine it getting any better. Within six months I had hit another new plateau of elation. This has happened to me several times in my sobriety. This is the most wonderful deal in the whole world for me.

This program is truly one of dreams. I have learned to build relationships with people. I have learned to share my innermost fears and secrets with others and have been comforted and have grown as a result. I have developed lifelong friendships and can relate to people on a level deeper than I could ever have hoped for before. I have experienced what true, deep, profound, unrestricted love is really like. This is the very first time I have ever felt these emotions.

Today I have a 13-year-old who has never seen me drunk or loaded. One Christmas, I wanted to buy him the most appropriate toy, so I asked him who his hero was. Without missing a beat, he turned and looked me right in the eyes and said, "You are, Daddy." That blew me away.

My older son moved in with me, and I had to work the Twelve Steps and the principles of the program in our relationship. He once looked me in my eyes and said, "You've ruined my life." All I could say to him was "Son, I might have made you sick, but I can't make you better. I haven't had a drink in over 10 years. I'm doing the best I can, and all I can do is give you what I've been given."

Last Father's Day, my son gave me a card. He is now back at college after being thrown out of school for drug and alcohol use six years ago. He is doing well and told me how proud he is of me.

Thank God for C.A., for teaching me how to regain my children's respect—that it isn't about telling them my great intentions, it's about showing them through my actions.

Thank you, C.A. Thank you to my sponsor and his wife, and to my wife and children. I believe God has operated through all these people and this program to give me the most wonderful life imaginable. If it was there for me, it is there for anybody who wants it, anyone willing to follow a few simple suggestions.

May God bless you and keep you always. May your bottom be so deep that you will put the shovel down and realize the only way out is by taking the Steps.

10

DOWNWARD SLIDE

His unmanageability took him to places he thought he'd never go; recovery brought him back.

Many people say they got high because of something that happened to them in their lives. I used simply because I liked the way it made me feel. I could not say that I didn't have clothes on my back or food on the table, because my parents both had excellent jobs and were good providers. My dad wrote a daily column for the largest newspaper in the state, and my mother had a well-paying state government job.

I can't say that I didn't feel like I belonged, because I was always popular in school. I played every sport, was in the chorus and drama club, always had a girlfriend, and was even president of the student council one year. I was a natural-born leader, and people seemed to like me. So I can't say that the reason I used drugs and alcohol was that I didn't fit in—because I did.

When I was growing up, the Serenity Prayer was on the wall in our bathroom. I remember going to visit Mom at the local mental hospital a couple of times when I was a kid. She went there to "rest" because of her "nerves." After my mother had died and I was around one year sober, I found an A.A. book while going through her estate. When I asked my father about it, he told me she was a member of A.A. I never knew it because it just wasn't talked about in those days. He had quit drinking when I was very young, but Mom never stopped.

I started getting high when I was 13 years old. I was busted at age 15 along with several others for felonious possession of a controlled substance with intent to sell. But I got out of it because my dad knew the right people, and since I was a juvenile, it was off my record by the time I turned 16.

I moved out on my 16th birthday and rented a house with some of the older kids from my neighborhood. I still went to school, mainly so I could sell marijuana to support myself. I would go to class and take the tests, and always managed to do well enough to make passing marks. In my senior year of high school, even though I had passing grades, they would not graduate me because I had missed too many days. I went to a local university, took my graduate equivalency degree, and got a scholarship to go to college because of Dad's military service.

By the end of my first semester in college, I was banned from all of the girls' dorms as well as all of the fraternity and sorority houses on campus. My grade point average was 0.001 because I had majored in "partying." I had to withdraw from school so I wouldn't lose my scholarship. I went back to a two-year school and got an associate degree in liberal arts.

With my college degree in hand, I went out into the world and got a job cleaning carpets. I was a good employee and supervisor and soon became a manager. Then I hurt my back and was out on worker's comp for a year and a half. I went to the chiropractor three times a week, got my pain pills, and collected a check every week. That was fine with me, and I milked it as long as possible. What could be better for an addict?

I was sent to vocational rehabilitation because there was no way I'd ever be able to clean carpets for a living again. I got a job with a local building supply company in sales. After three months, they promoted me to management.

I was still using drugs, mainly smoking pot and drinking beer, but managed to make it to work every day. My best friend came back from college and moved into my house. I didn't know it, but he had become an IV drug user. That was something I said I would never do because I had seen it destroy my brother. Then, the very first night my friend moved in, I started shooting up cocaine.

My addiction began to take over my life. I was still a workaholic, but I began to leave bills unpaid, bounced a check every once in a while, and even showed up late for work a few times.

One night while I was trying to score drugs, someone ripped me off. I got my throat cut when I tried to get my money back. As soon as I got out of the hospital, I went straight to the dealer to get some cocaine. A normal person would have stopped using dope, but I was an addict.

I met a girl at work, and she soon became pregnant with our child. Around the same time, my best friend died of a drug overdose. When I went to the funeral, I looked at him lying in the casket and swore I would never put another needle in my arm. I never did: no Twelve Steps, no treatment, no Higher Power—I just stopped on my own.

My girlfriend and I got married, and she gave birth to a beautiful baby boy. I was there when he was born and even cut the umbilical cord. I swore that I was going to be the best father that there ever was because I loved my son.

Somewhere around two years after my son was born, I was still off the needle but indulging in other substances at every opportunity. My drinking had also increased. One evening, I went over to pick up my son at the new babysitter's and discovered that her husband was an old friend of mine. He invited me in the house to get high on what turned out to be crack cocaine. Immediately I knew I had found my drug of choice. It wasn't as bad as needles, right? I went back to his house several times that night to get more. I had to have it.

From there, I am sure you all know the story. I'll just give you the highlights. Pawnshops, bad neighborhoods at 4 a.m., missed work, bad checks, final notices, utility shut-offs, eviction notices, going to score in the middle of the night while my precious little son was asleep—just to mention a few of the things that happened in active addiction.

In August 1998, my son was put in foster care for neglect. Basically, neglect meant that he was left home alone while my wife and I went out to score. The judge ordered me to go to five meetings a week and do anything the social worker planned for me in my "reunification" plan. My wife and I were separated, and she went into a halfway house.

I liked going to meetings. People would listen to me spout off about how I really was a good father and all of the other delusions I had spun for myself, smile at me and tell me to keep coming back. My master plan was to go to meetings, get my piece of paper signed for the social worker, and all would be well. I would stay clean for a while, my wife would come back, my son would come home, and we would live happily ever after. An addict with a plan.

I relapsed a few times trying to work my selective version of the Twelve Steps. I even wrote a paper on how God could keep me clean, took it to a meeting, and asked them if I could read it out loud. My sponsor (whom I called every two weeks to inform him how I had already done the first Three Steps on my own) said we'd save it for the end of the meeting. They ran out of time before I got to read it. Imagine that.

As a result of my actions, Child Protective Services had me check into outpatient rehab. My counselor said he was going to keep me clean no matter what I did. My weekly schedule was two parenting classes, three nights of intensive outpatient therapy, five meetings, two scheduled drug screens, and one random screen. I got to see my son for a half hour every other week under supervision. I also had to keep a job and be able to provide a "suitable living environment" if I ever wanted to bring my little boy home again.

Finally, I had managed 30 days of clean drug screens. I went for my Monday visit with the social worker. She informed me I would be tested on Tuesday and that they were going to rush the results. If it came up clean, I could have my son eight hours on Saturday, totally unsupervised. If it came up dirty, I would never see him again.

Normally on Mondays I went to a 5:30 meeting, a 6:45 meeting, and an 8 o'clock meeting at a local clubhouse. On that particular Monday, I could just head on home as I had enough meeting sheets signed for the social worker. On the way home, I stopped at the store and bought one beer.

That night I smoked endless amounts of crack. But something different happened to me. I couldn't get high. No matter how much I sucked on that stem, it didn't work anymore. I peeked out the blinds, hid in the closet, crawled around on the floor looking for the one I had dropped even though I still had some. The thing that really hit me, though, was the tears rolling down my face because I knew I would never see my son again.

I loved my son with all of my heart. I was not a bad person. But no matter who or what I thought I was, I couldn't stop smoking crack. With full knowledge that I would lose him forever, I still got high. The guilt, shame, and misery of addiction swept over me like never before.

When I woke up the next morning, I had absolutely no hope whatsoever. I had to take that drug screen, and there was no way out of it. There was nothing left for me in my life. Cocaine was my master.

I called the drug counselor, the foster parents, the court-appointed guardian, and the few people I knew in the program. Every single one of them had the same answer. What are you going to do differently? I had lost my son forever and could not stay clean for him, so how's about doing it for myself? I had nothing to lose.

I took my drug screen and then went to a meeting to get another white newcomer chip. When I walked up, this lady whom I had seen in the meetings whispered in my ear as she gave me the chip, "This is the last one." It scared me, but somehow I knew she was right. I never got high again.

I chaired my first meeting at three days clean and sober and got a sponsor. He told me that service work was the backbone of recovery, so I became involved at every level. Since then I have been asked to serve in every service position at every level. I became involved, at his suggestion, in the online meetings and through that have had an opportunity to make new friends from all over the world.

My sponsor worked the program of Cocaine Anonymous with me. Every week I went to his house, and we worked the Twelve Steps together. In working Step One with a sponsor, I finally understood my own personal experience with powerlessness and unmanageability.

Powerlessness was about the physical allergy and the mental obsession. The physical allergy means that once I take that first hit of any mind-altering substance, I can't stop. For me it as simple as that one beer that I drank the day before I took that drug screen. For me it was as clear as putting away the needle for several years, and the minute I smoked crack, I was right back where I left off, only worse.

It is easy to see the physical unmanageability in active addiction. We all have our stories about that: lost jobs, broken families, all our possessions ending up in a pawnshop, etc. What I didn't understand, but had experienced, was the unmanageability of my spirit. The total misery and hopelessness that I felt the last time I used is something that I never want to feel again.

It was only through working the program of Cocaine Anonymous that I connected with a Power greater than myself that removed my addiction to cocaine, alcohol, and all other mind-altering substances. If you are an addict like me, walk, swim, fly, crawl, or run to the closest C.A. meeting you can find. Get yourself a sponsor, work the Steps, read the literature, and get to know the people in the Fellowship.

It has worked for me. I wouldn't trade my life today with anybody. My son has lived with me for over five years now. He's been to so many meetings with me, he even knows the Third Step Prayer and the Serenity Prayer by heart. Today I own a house and am married to a beautiful, loving wife, with over 10 years clean and sober. The Promises have come true in a way I never thought possible, thanks to the program of Cocaine Anonymous.

11

CALL COCAINE ANONYMOUS, WE CAN HELP

The C.A. helpline directed him to his first meeting. Through working the Steps, he has replaced a cocaine high with a spiritual connection.

Some in the program call me a high-bottom addict, but I sure didn't feel very high when I bottomed out in the spring of 1990. I never went to jail, never lost a job, and never had a DUI, but when I walked into my first meeting of Cocaine Anonymous, I was physically, emotionally, and spiritually broken. Cocaine had taken me to a dark and demoralizing place from which I didn't know how to escape.

It wasn't always that way. For years cocaine and other mind-altering substances did for me what I couldn't do for myself. Cocaine, alcohol, and other drugs made me feel confident, important, and more comfortable in a world where I often felt like a stranger in a strange land.

Of course, like many other cocaine addicts, my using habits didn't begin with cocaine. I began my using career drinking alcohol and smoking pot during high school. Then I graduated to acid, mushrooms, Quaaludes, and just about anything else that was available.

Somewhere in the haze of the late 1970s, during my junior year of high school, I bought my first cocaine. I was washing dishes at a restaurant and disco and discovered that a waitress there was selling the stuff. I bought a quarter gram for $30, and she handed me a small brown vial with a little bit of white powder in the bottom. I was shocked at how little a quarter gram was. I figured it must be really potent stuff.

I took home my little stash of cocaine, looked at it for a while, played with it on a little mirror, drew a tiny little line, and snorted it up my nose. Then I waited for the big rush. Nothing happened. I called a druggie friend and told her that I had snorted some cocaine. After a while, I convinced myself that I felt high and tried to impress her with talk of my newfound wonder drug. This friend would soon become the person with whom I first smoked and mainlined cocaine.

That first quarter gram lasted me three weeks. In the coming years, a quarter gram would last me no more than a few minutes.

In the next year, I grew to love cocaine. Still in high school, I got a better paying job and found a connection that sold cocaine cheaper. I also found that cocaine helped me with my second favorite pastime—women. Cocaine made me feel bold, confident, and sexual.

During college, I used and dealt cocaine. It was during the punk/New Wave scene, and life was good. I was having a blast bingeing on cocaine, selling it to friends at the bars, and using it to keep me awake late at night during my studies. Coming from a long line of functional addicts and alcoholics, I managed to graduate from college with honors, but my cocaine use began to turn dark near the end of college and got even worse after that.

At around age 23 or 24, I went beyond being a social or even a hard user. The physical craving got so bad near the end that my preference was to be entirely alone while using. I become the person described in *Who is a Cocaine Addict?* I would take a hit in the closet, walk into the living room, stare out the blinds for a few minutes to see who might be coming, then walk back into the closet for another hit. I would repeat this little dance for hours until I ran out.

I remember one incident that really shook me, but not enough to get sober. I was working in a restaurant while waiting to begin a student teaching assignment in preparation for becoming a high school teacher. I gave a coworker a ride home and ended up drinking and snorting crystal with him, his sister, and several of her friends. I had no idea these kids attended the school where I would begin teaching just days later. To my astonishment, one of those kids came up to me at school and asked me if I wanted to go across the street to get high with him and some other students. I was mortified. I didn't get high that day, but I didn't get sober, either.

My last day using came several months later. I hadn't used cocaine in months, thanks to my alcohol and marijuana maintenance program. During the school day, the mental obsession to use entered my mind, and I couldn't shake it. Immediately after classes ended, I bought a crack pipe and headed for the dealer's house. Later that afternoon I took my first hit of cocaine, and the tidal wave of the physical addiction swept over me. I quickly rocked up most of the cocaine, hiding various stashes around the house in case my fiancée should come home and find my stash.

Because my cocaine lockjaw had kicked in, I could barely put together an articulate sentence when she came in the door. After a few minutes, I heard her scream as she found the first stash of rock hidden under the bed. She began crying and told me she would leave for good if I didn't give her the pipe and the rest of the cocaine. She seemed serious. I thought about her proposal for about 30 seconds and then told her she would not be getting my cocaine. She was horrified and started packing. While she packed, which seemed to take hours, all I could think was, "What is taking her so long to leave? I haven't had a hit in 30 minutes." She finally left, allowing me to finish smoking my cocaine and then drink myself to sleep.

When I came to, I realized I had traded my fiancée for a few hits off the crack pipe. It was a brief moment of clarity, followed by an opportunity. A public service announcement came on TV stating, "If you have a problem with cocaine, call Cocaine Anonymous. We can help." I wrote down the number. I believe that moment was necessary for me to take that first step into the rooms of recovery. From what I've observed, the window of opportunity and willingness is often brief, and if I had not acted upon it immediately, it may have snapped shut. I went to my first C.A. meeting the next day.

The meeting was at a dingy little halfway house, and there were about seven or eight people in attendance. The first person I saw could tell I was new, so he gave me a big smile, stuck out his hand, welcomed me, and told me his name. That man became my first sponsor, my roommate for six years, and one of my dearest friends to this day.

After the others had introduced themselves, it was my turn. For the first time, the truth I had known for so long fell out of my mouth: "My name is _____, and I'm an addict." Admitting to this group of people that I was an addict was my first surrender, and a huge weight lifted from my shoulders.

I believe that, like spiritual experiences, there are two types of First Step experiences: the educational variety and the burning-bush type. I've had both, but at that first meeting, I had a visceral, gut-wrenching epiphany that I was powerless over my addiction and could not stay sober on my own.

I grabbed onto the program like a drowning man grabs onto a life preserver. I attended a meeting almost every day and three on Friday nights because that was payday, and the beginnings of the weekends were always tough for me. I also went to dinner and coffee with other addicts after meetings, did service work, and began to work on the Steps. After a month, my first sponsor nominated me to chair the halfway house meeting. That early service commitment was one of the things that kept me sober.

One of the events that sealed my desire to stay clean occurred just before my 60 days. I was told C.A. would be holding a world convention in my hometown and that I should go. I was reluctant to attend, not knowing many people, but I was reminded that in order to stay sober, I needed to get involved, so I did. I spent $20 I thought I couldn't afford to attend the banquet and speaker meeting.

I walked into the room not knowing where to sit and found an empty seat at a table of members from out of town. They were all cordial until someone asked me how much time I had. When I told them 50-some days, their demeanor changed. All of a sudden, I was the center of attention because I was the newcomer. They gave me suggestions, phone numbers, and encouragement. At the end of the meal, when tickets were drawn to win the centerpiece, they gave it to me, even though my number wasn't drawn.

Let me say this: no gesture toward helping the newcomer is unimportant or too small. The smallest gesture or effort can help keep the newcomer sober for one more day—and that day might be the day the newcomer finally "gets it."

The evening got even better when I witnessed my first sobriety countdown. They started with 25 years of sobriety, and an old-timer stepped up to the stage, said a few words, and was handed a book that most people at the convention had signed. When they started counting down by months and got to 30 days, I stood up, feeling proud at my accomplishment, but humbled at how many people had so much more sobriety.

The excitement built to a fever pitch as they counted down to 24 hours. A frightened young woman stood up and was ushered to the stage by people in the crowd. I found myself, like all the others in attendance, cheering wildly, clapping and chanting, "Keep coming back, keep coming back!" It was electric. The man with 25 years hugged her and gave her the signed book. Ten years later, that same woman, with 10 years of sobriety, took the stage at the C.A. World Convention and handed another young woman with 24 hours a "Big Book" signed by hundreds of recovering addicts. That's the miracle of passing it on. After the countdown, we formed a huge circle to close the meeting. It was during the countdown, and especially during the closing prayer, arm in arm with hundreds of other addicts, that I had what I consider my first spiritual experience in sobriety. I felt the presence of God coursing through all of us in that room.

I realized two things that night. First, even though I had only 50-some days of sobriety, I had something to offer the person with 50-some hours. Second, I wanted what these people had and was willing to go to any lengths to get it.

It wasn't easy staying sober at first. There were many days I didn't think I would make it. At those times, I did what had been suggested to me by members of the Fellowship: I would go to a meeting, call another addict, pick up the literature, or pray—a lot. Many a rough night required that I do all of these things.

I also learned something about relationships in my first year of recovery. The key is that the recovery must always come before the relationship. Without recovery, I was incapable of engaging in a healthy relationship; and relationships, more than any other factor in that first year, almost got me loaded several times.

I heard a member of the Fellowship say that the weeks, months, and years had flown by, but on some days it had seemed damn near impossible to stay sober. For me, in early sobriety, the key was surviving those few hellish days—one day at a time. But those days passed. I discovered that if you can survive that handful of difficult days, a miracle awaits on the other side. My favorite tired old cliché saying in recovery is, "Don't give up five minutes before the miracle happens."

After waiting far too long and feeling sure I was on the way to relapse again, I asked a man whose program I respected to help me with the Fourth Step. I had been doing the One-Two-Three-Step shuffle, and as a result, my spiritual house was not clean. We did the Fourth through Seventh Steps immediately that day. As a result, I was able to begin to shed the guilt, shame, anger, and remorse that were crowding out the conscious contact with my Higher Power that I need to stay sober.

After that day I continued to work through the Steps, made my amends, and attempted to promptly admit my wrongs and improve my conscious contact with God. My life continued to get better—not perfect, but better.

Somewhere during that time, a miracle happened. One day I realized that I no longer had the obsession to use. I can't pinpoint the moment when the obsession left me, but I know I was sober and working a program when it did. It was sometime around my Fifth Step experience.

Near my seventh year, I reached another crossroad in my recovery. All was wonderful in my life. I had a gotten married to a beautiful woman I met in recovery, had a child, and had just completed a master's degree. As happens with some of us when life gets busy, I was hanging out on the edge of the program. I still attended a few meetings and had the same friends, but I was not sponsoring anyone, nor was I doing any service work.

One night while playing volleyball, I felt something tear inside my chest. I attempted to walk out of the gym, but there was an incredible pain in my shoulder and back, and I was having trouble breathing. A teammate drove me to the emergency room, where the doctors discovered that I had a collapsed lung, a potentially fatal injury. The surgeons had to operate twice. After 12 days, my lung had finally healed, and I was sent home.

During my time in the hospital and at home recovering, many family members and friends from the program came to see me. One member of the Fellowship even mowed my lawn. I was overwhelmed. Something occurred to me during those days. I realized that I was one of the most blessed people on the planet and that I needed to start giving back again.

Shortly after that, I joined the committee for a World Service Convention and began an incredible three-year journey with a group of dedicated addicts. I picked up many other commitments over the next few years at the local, Area, and World level. To this day, I continue to do service work and love it (most of the time). I've also discovered that service work is an excellent way to work on my character defects. Nothing brings out my ego, pride, judgment, and self-righteousness like dealing with numerous personalities, many of whom disagree with me on a variety of issues.

Perhaps the greatest gifts I have received over the past few years are my relationships with my family and with my sponsees. I sponsor a dozen or so men, some with under a year and some with double-digit sobriety. They help me stay sober and teach me so much. By working with them, I have become a little less selfish and have grown as a person. It's very hard to work the Steps with a sponsee and not examine one's own shortcomings and defects.

I've heard it said that alcoholics and addicts are some of the most spiritual people on earth, but the problem is that we often choose the wrong spirit. Before I got sober, I sought the spirit in the straw, the pipe, and the needle. Today, another spirit guides me—the spirit of God and of Cocaine Anonymous. I have replaced a cocaine high with a spiritual connection that comes from working the Twelve Steps and working with others. I am truly grateful to those who came before me in this Fellowship and stuck around to carry this message to me, so that I might get sober and carry it to others.

Today I continue to be an active member of the Fellowship. I attend meetings, actively engage in service work, sponsor other addicts, and continue to carry the message of recovery.

On many occasions, I wonder what I have done to deserve all that I have received. I give back to C.A. because it is my responsibility to carry this message and an honor to do so, but I don't know if I will ever be able to give back what I've been given. I'm just an addict among other addicts, and what I see every day amazes me. In Cocaine Anonymous, I see God's work all around. We are men and women who, prior to Twelve-Step recovery, had been hopeless, often homeless or institutionalized. We were dying. Now we in recovery are men and women righting the wrongs of our past; regaining the respect of friends, peers, and colleagues; thinking about the welfare of others; paying our bills; and acting as good parents, spouses, and responsible members of our communities. How can one not be humbled by this vision? Like my life, it is a true miracle.

12

FINALLY HOME

Blaming God for his father's death, this addict drank and drugged his way through life. Now, through C.A. and God's help, he is free from the misery, terror and pain of being a using addict.

I come from an upper-working-class family—meaning my dad had a job. We moved from north of the English countryside down south to the coast when I was four months old. We were poor, and the family survived the best it could. My memories of early childhood are dim. My mum stayed home, my dad taught in schools, and we had a dog called Blackie; that was it, really. Unbeknown to me, my father had been very ill since the age of 19 with a rare kidney disease. He later developed Crohn's disease, cancer, and mental problems. As a consequence of this, his diet became pureed mush, and we didn't do too much as a family.

We all began to suffer, or at least that's what this addict thought. No father at football, boring food, no laughter, no parties, no holidays, just the realization something wasn't quite right. Men came in white coats, and there was talk of electric shock treatment, straitjackets, and insanity. At around nine or 10 years old, I began to put my hands in electric sockets to see what shock treatment felt like. It was horrible! Why were they doing this to my dad? Where was he going when he left the house? What was happening? No one would answer my questions. Fear gripped me, and I felt terrible. I was alone and isolated—a bad place to be at 10 years old. I began to find pills in my father's pockets, and I took them. I stole money. I hung with orphans because they never went on about their parents. I began to shut down emotionally and struggled to communicate at all.

After numerous hospitals and specialists, my father went away and never came back. I was put with a friend whose religious father locked me in cupboards and tried to beat me, so I ran away. Mother would phone occasionally with news of my father, most of the time about failed operations and a steady decline. He was about to die, but of course no one said this to me.

Following my father's death, I cranked up the odds—weed, pills, speed, and acid, with no particular favourite apart from more.

I was done with God; He had killed my dad, and there was no going back, ever! My descent into hell had begun, and I didn't even know it.

School became a chore, so hanging out and skipping lessons became the norm. I dealt to get extra cash and smoked a lot. After being thrown out of school for various reasons, I left for London. I returned home only to borrow and steal to get what I needed. I scraped through college and dreamed of fame and fortune. I began to sell clothes that I designed to hip shops. I was rewarded with cocaine and never looked back—this was the drug I had been looking for.

Success equalled cocaine, and therefore cocaine meant success: what a concept. For almost two decades, this is what motivated me. Cocaine woke me up and let me talk to girls. I played and worked hard. I found myself in France and Italy, still using. I thought I was in control despite several disturbing events—being shot at, mugged, jumping out of windows. I took all of this in stride. Returning to the U.K., I worked in record shops and made a few things, but basically I survived by dealing. Even as a dealer, I fell short and never seemed to make any money. It had never occurred to me not to get high on my supply.

I met a nurse and married her; surely she would save me. We used any and all drugs, including some she stole from work. Again, I seemed to have fallen on my feet, but it did not last. I left after a few months; the cocaine was more important than the marriage, and she kept going on all the time anyway. I needed some peace, so I moved in with a heroin addict who didn't like coke.

Isolated with another addict and with no work to speak of, things got worse. I was attacked and beaten up. With my health declining rapidly, I was still in full denial, and blamed anyone and everything.

How could it be my fault? Heroin became light relief and reality a distant blur. There were court appearances, driving offences and cautions, and I still did not stop using. How could I? Debts mounted, and work stopped. I lived by theft and pathetic dealing; no big stuff, just grams and pills, no ounces or bags. This was mere existence, scrabbling in the dirt for scraps and being beaten into submission. I was burnt to the ground. I could not go on, but I could not stop. I had arrived in hell.

I phoned an old customer who had stopped using. Could he help me? Well, yes, he could. In the summer of 1992, I stopped. What a relief to admit the complete and utter defeat of being an addict. We went straight to a smoky meeting of another Twelve-Step Fellowship. I had arrived in recovery; these people weren't addicts, but just maybe they could help me? They laughed, they shared, they cried, and they let me in! The first 90 days were scary and a blur; the suggestions, points, hints, experience, and advice were all too much. I pressed on. No God, no Steps, no sponsor, no beer, no coke, no clue—but a tiny bit of hope, a glimmer of things to come, and that persistent mantra: keep coming back.

Gradually, I began to thaw out. I spoke to people; there was no mention of drugs by them but lots of drug talk by me. They never said a thing. What love, what tolerance they showed me! But my feeling of uselessness did not recede, and I couldn't really make friends. I finally asked for help: What should I do?

A man informed me that he could now sponsor me, and we would see how we got on. Carrying out instructions (unless drugs were involved) was groundbreaking stuff for this addict. We started the Steps, me, my sponsor, and God—what a team. I knew it would be all right because my sponsor told me so, and I believed him. This was progress indeed.

At about that same time, I began to share about drugs in their meetings. People mostly shrugged and didn't comment, but one lady approached me. "I have the very thing for you," she said. "Come and do the share at C.A. on Saturday. You will like it there, I'm sure." So I went to C.A.

Some of my friends from the other meetings were there. Why hadn't they told me about this place? The coffee tasted good, the welcome was fantastic, and the stories were the same as mine. I had arrived at the final destination: God had brought me to C.A., and I was home. I cried for days at the relief of finally belonging somewhere. I dived into service and made tea, greeted, became a secretary, all those things we do at meetings—I joined in. Life began to take shape as the Steps began to change me and I became willing to change. My belief strengthened as time went by. Through prayer and meditation, I quietly found a better relationship with my God.

I became a GSR (Group Service Representative) and went to Area. It was scary stuff again. I made a fool of myself, put my feet everywhere, and learned to promptly admit it when I was wrong. I served on Public Information and Hospitals & Institutions Committees, going to prisons and treatment centres. I even ventured abroad to be of service.

I did what I was told, and my life expanded. I got a business so I could pay my bills. My mother died, and I didn't use—in fact, I got married two days after burying her. I now have three stepchildren who teach me stuff daily.

Twelve years ago I wanted to die every time I awoke, and escape seemed impossible for an addict like me. Cocaine Anonymous has shown me the way and has never let me down. The Higher Power of my understanding keeps me clean, and I live life to the full every day. Taking people through the Steps helps me and may even help them. Each day is as joyful as I decide to make it, and I am truly happy most days. God has showered me with such wonderful friends, and everything is so fantastic. With God's help and His grace, I now live free from the misery, terror, and pain of being a using addict.

13

AN ATTITUDE OF GRATITUDE

Practicing gratitude totally turned her attitude around, and looking for the good in her life became a reflex.

"Help me. Please help me," I sobbed, as I lay in a crumpled heap on the floor. I wasn't talking to anyone in particular, since I didn't believe in God. I had been crawling the grungy beige shag carpet for hours, looking desperately for some cocaine I knew I'd never dropped in the first place, when the dawn started creeping in around the blinds, and it struck me how pathetic my life had become. I was broke, unemployed, being evicted, and so skeletally thin that a friend said she was afraid I was going to die. Worst of all was the utter desolation I felt inside. Cocaine had been keeping those feelings at bay, but coming down, it was all too painfully clear what a mess I'd made of my life.

I didn't know it then, but that morning in 1987 was my moment of surrender. I have been clean and sober ever since.

I am the only child of a loving, decent, middle-class family. There was no alcohol, drug, or other abuse in our home, just a strong sense of how important it was to say and do the right thing. My parents were proud of my good grades, but the other kids teased me for being smart. In response, I became painfully shy; books, TV, and movies were my refuge. Becoming an addict and alcoholic certainly wasn't what I had in mind. I wanted to be a famous actress or a writer, something dramatic and exciting. I mostly dreamed of a day when I could feel like I fit in with the rest of the world.

That day finally came in junior high, when I started drinking and smoking pot. At first I didn't like the taste and did it just for the effect—and how I loved the effect! For once, I felt comfortable in my own skin, and everybody seemed to like me. Drugs and alcohol took away my loneliness and filled up what had felt like a gaping hole in my soul. Before long, I found it difficult to live without them.

The occasional weekend party soon escalated to getting high every day. It was the 1970s, and sex, drugs, and rock-and-roll ruled. After my first keg party, I lost my virginity to a guy I'd just met, the first of a long string of promiscuous acts while under the influence. Speed and psychedelic drugs soon also became part of the picture, and I was willing to try almost anything to get high.

I began living a dual life—the party girl with my friends but still the good girl at home. My parents became suspicious and searched my room, where they found my journals, birth control pills, beer, pot, and paraphernalia. They tried to force me to quit, but I only became more defiant and determined to get out on my own. I graduated with honors and became a legal secretary, the highest paying job I could get without college.

The day after my 18th birthday, I moved to a place where there was always a neighbor willing to buy liquor or help find drugs. The party was on, big time. Since I worked in the legal profession, I used to joke about being Ms. Legal by day, Ms. Illegal by night. My disease was progressing rapidly.

I didn't use cocaine until shortly after I turned 21. Coke had always scared me because it was a "hard drug," but it was love at first snort. Cocaine made me feel good in a way I'd never experienced before. Initially, I was able to control my usage, but it soon escalated out of control.

I decided to make my fortune as a cocaine dealer after it became too difficult to get up the next morning and go to work. Two regular customers introduced me to freebasing. After my first hit, all I felt was warm and slightly nauseated. So I did what any good drug addict would do: I said, "Gimme another one." That second hit sealed my fate. It gave me exactly the sensation I'd been seeking for so many years, and I wondered how I'd ever lived without such a wonderful thing in my life.

The more coke I did, the more I drank. After a margarita binge, I found myself drinking straight triple sec at 7 a.m. That scared me because I thought only alcoholics drank in the morning, so I decided to quit drinking. I went through a horrible case of the DTs. After five months of not drinking, I felt I'd proven I wasn't an alcoholic, so I did what any good alcoholic would do: I started drinking again. Trouble was, I could no longer hold my liquor, and one night I awoke vomiting in my own bed. It scared me that I could have choked to death in my sleep, so once again I decided to go easy on the alcohol.

I soon reached the end of the road as a coke dealer, after too many fronts and using too much of what I was supposed to be selling. My former dealing partner was murdered, and cocaine became harder to find, so I started letting others deal out of my house. My entire existence revolved around cocaine—getting it, using it up, and then getting more. Even when I had cocaine, it was no longer doing the job, and I was starting to combine it with other drugs like nitrous oxide in an effort to recapture the intense high I'd gotten when I first started freebasing.

My health was starting to suffer, and I was losing it mentally. I rarely bathed and had no clean clothes. Dirty dishes were stacked several layers deep around the kitchen, and I had tacked sheets and blankets up over all the windows to ease my paranoia. The bills and shut-off notices were piling up, and my landlord began eviction proceedings—which was ironic, since I used to do evictions for a living.

I halfheartedly tried to get sober twice on my own, just to prove I could do it. Both times, Friday night rolled around, and I ended up using again.

In either desperation or defiance, I finally told my mother that I was doing cocaine. My parents did their best to help but only ended up enabling me. After some research, they decided to practice tough love and brought me a written ultimatum: go to treatment, or live on the street. My mother handed me some stationery and postage stamps and said, "Let us know where you end up." Now, that got my attention! I knew deep down that something had to change, so I reluctantly agreed to go to treatment. I didn't know what I was getting myself into, but I wanted out of the hell my life had become.

My things were sent to storage while I did my best to put off the inevitable, staying in the empty house so I could use just one more time. After that last use, I had my moment of surrender. I'd finally had enough.

In treatment, I was introduced to Cocaine Anonymous. When someone read "snorting or smoking any white speck from the floor when we ran out," I knew I was home. While I was none too keen on giving up all other mind-altering substances, the folks at the C.A. meeting seemed to be having quite a good time without them. I realized I couldn't be convinced the program didn't work until I actually tried it.

The fellowship aspect of the program immediately won me over. The Steps, however, intimidated me. I could deal with the First Step but not those that mentioned God, a Higher Power, or spirituality. I didn't understand then that the Steps are a recipe for a spiritual awakening, and they're in a specific order for good reason. I'd thought God was simply a crutch for weak people, and I refused to see myself as weak. At 11 days sober, I wrote in my journal about not wanting to force myself to believe in any God and not wanting to relinquish control of myself to anything external. I added, "I have made too much progress with me at the helm to want to leave the bridge!" I then made the kind of decision only a toxic mind can make: to use my own will power as my Higher Power. Talk about denial—I couldn't see that my best thinking had landed me in treatment.

Giving up the struggle gradually allowed me to become as open-minded and willing as possible. In just a few weeks I went from being an atheist to having a working faith in a Higher Power, although my path to that faith was somewhat unconventional. My cat had disappeared, and I was frantic. After looking for her to no avail, I decided to pray about it. I asked God to please bring her back and promised to treat her better if He did. The very next morning, the doorbell rang, and there was a little girl with my cat in her arms. I was overjoyed and thought to myself, "This God stuff works!" I've since learned that my Higher Power is not some sort of cosmic vending machine, where I drop in a prayer and out pops whatever I want, but that experience was just what I needed at the time.

At a few months sober, I was consumed by anger and regret over the past and realized I needed to do a Fourth Step. It was time to get a sponsor, so I asked an assertive, no-nonsense woman. Frankly, she scared me to death, but I knew she wouldn't let me lie my way through the process. Once we started working together, however, instead of scaring me into telling the truth, she provided a place where it was safe to do so.

In early sobriety, my thoughts were totally about me: what a piece of garbage I was and how my life sucked. When I started whining, my sponsor had me make a daily list of five things I was grateful for, and every day it had to be five different things. I started with the basics, like being grateful to be alive, but some days even that was a stretch. I was always happy to point out how the glass was half empty rather than half full. Learning to practice gratitude totally turned my attitude around, and looking for the good in my life soon became a reflex. I used to be baffled when I heard people say they were grateful to be an addict or an alcoholic, but now I understand, because without this disease I would never have been introduced to this wonderful program of recovery. I'm even grateful for the painful experiences in my recovery, because they afford me an opportunity for growth.

My sponsor and I went over the first three Steps before moving on to the Fourth, and she helped me develop a working relationship with a Higher Power of my own understanding. She let me know it was okay to let go of the image I had of a judgmental, punishing God and replace it with a God who is my ever-present best friend, unconditionally loving and supportive. For me the key was realizing God could be whatever I needed Him to be. I'm grateful C.A.

gives us the room to find a God of our own understanding, for I doubt I could have done it any other way.

When it came time to do my Fourth Step, my sponsor told me to find some place where I wouldn't be disturbed and to pray before I started writing, so that God would be in charge of what came out on the paper, not me. Writing my Fourth Step was very cathartic; it felt so good to dump what had been poisoning my spirit for so long. I had 17 pages of resentments alone! As good as it felt to vent about what everyone had done to me, it was incredibly enlightening to look at my part in the fourth column. I actually had a part in every one of those resentments. I began to see that I wasn't just a victim, I was a perpetrator—and that knowledge was the key to setting me free.

The Fifth Step was a turning point not just in my recovery but in my entire life. My sponsor asked questions to make sure I got everything off my chest and shared similar experiences so I knew I wasn't alone. She also had me look at what I'd done right and what good qualities I had. I felt so light and so free afterward, like a huge weight had been lifted from my shoulders. I'd spent most of my life not being able to look people in the eye, for fear they'd see what a horrible person I was. After my Fifth Step, I no longer felt like an awful person and could literally face the world for the first time. When I looked in the mirror afterward, I almost didn't recognize myself.

After my Fifth Step, my sponsor asked whom I resented most, and I said my mother. For years, our relationship had been strained at best. Toward the end of my using, I avoided seeing my parents because Mom and I always ended up in a fight. My sponsor told me to pray for my mother every day for two weeks. To say I balked is an understatement, but everything else my sponsor had suggested to that point had worked. Plus, as she put it, "Just try it for two weeks. What have you got to lose?"

As it turned out, what I had to lose was a big resentment. Mom and I now have a wonderfully loving relationship. If that isn't a miracle of recovery, I don't know what is. Thanks to that amazing experience, it is now much easier to look at my part and pray for the other person.

It was also interesting to look at how fearful I was and to begin the process of using faith to cure fear. Occasionally I still struggle with fear, including a perverse fear of truly being or having everything I want in life. I have more recently started asking God to help me refrain from self-defeating behaviors and attitudes, so that I may become the person He would have me be and that I desire to be.

When I trust in my Higher Power, do the footwork, and leave the results to God, things turn out much better. I love those words, "the courage to change." Change is scary, but necessary if I am to grow as a human being. I'm grateful that I have willingness to change today, and that I can get whatever courage I need from my Higher Power and this Fellowship.

I did well with Step Six but had a little trouble when I got to Seven. When I first started saying the Seventh Step Prayer, I added a list of which defects God should remove and in what order. Nothing seemed to be happening, until I realized that I wasn't being very humble if I was telling God what to do. As soon as I started saying the prayer without my laundry list attached, I started seeing and feeling the results.

My sponsor said Steps Six and Seven are a lifelong process, and that has proven true in my experience. When my defects become painful enough, I become willing to let God remove them—in His time, and in His way. I also began asking God every morning to help me be honest, tolerant, and truly loving toward the rest of the world and Him. I learned that it's actually much easier on me when I approach everyone and everything with an attitude of love and tolerance.

When it came to my Eighth Step, I again prayed before I put pen to paper. I was astonished when I wrote the name of a former next-door neighbor whose boyfriend I had stolen when I was 18. He moved from her house into mine, resulting in numerous drunken brawls and property damage. I had never looked at my part until that moment, when I realized I had started the whole thing. I made a written amends to her, since I didn't feel safe seeing her in person. By then, the man was married to someone else, but I thought my motives were pure enough that I could make a direct amends to him. As soon as we saw each other, however, all our old feelings resurfaced, and we began another affair. My sponsor told me that making amends isn't just about apologizing; it's about changing the behavior. Obviously, I hadn't changed the behavior, and I quickly became very spiritually sick. I broke off the affair when I realized I had to if I ever hoped to stay sober.

Step Ten helps keep my side of the street clean. Whenever I'm angry or upset, I love reading about the Tenth Step. It helps me regain my perspective, so I can see my part and forgive others for theirs when necessary.

Working Step Eleven has been incredibly rewarding. My conscious contact with God grows stronger all the time. I am learning to trust the process and to listen to my gut without my head intervening.

I love Step Twelve because it helps get me out of myself. I started service work at a few months sober and have been blessed to be of service at the Group, District, Area, and/or World levels ever since. As a result, I have a great respect for the Traditions and the power of the group conscience. Being a sponsor is the most rewarding part of the Step for me—there's nothing like seeing the lights come on in the eyes of a newcomer. I try not to tell my sponsees what to do; instead, I share what I did, suggest that they try it, and see if it works for them. Sponsees are truly a blessing; they keep me focused on the Steps and give me an opportunity to pass on what was so freely given to me.

At about seven years sober, I learned the importance of not resting on my laurels. I succumbed to the temptation to live a so-called normal life. I cut back to only one meeting a week, stopped praying, and had only minimal contact with other recovering addicts. I quickly became very spiritually sick, and although I didn't want to drink or use, I wanted to drive into a brick wall to end my pain. One of my sponsees gently told me I no longer had what she wanted, and I realized I needed to pick up the tools of the program again. Thankfully, they started working immediately. I vowed that I would never again stop working on my recovery on a daily basis, and I've stuck to that vow.

I also try to remember that I'm not doing anyone any good by keeping my problems to myself because I somehow feel my length of sobriety means I have to look and sound a certain way. The truth is, life still happens, and sometimes I am a bit of a mess—and sharing that I'm working through it sober is actually the best way to carry the message that the program does work.

Thank God I jumped back into the program with both feet when I did, for there were soon tough times in my recovery. I learned my father had lung cancer and had only six months to live. I curled up in a fetal position, heartbroken and sobbing, saying my simplest prayer, "Help me, please help me." That time I knew exactly who I was talking to, and He answered. Moments later I got a call from a friend in the program who'd lost his own father. God gave me just what I needed, just when I needed it most.

As the reality of the situation set in, I realized I had a clear choice between anger and acceptance: anger had the power to kill me, whereas acceptance had the power to save me. I could either look at God as the One who gave my father a terminal illness or the One who was going to help me get through it. Although I desperately wanted my father to survive, I didn't want to pray for a specific result and risk destroying my faith if I didn't get it. I knew God wouldn't give me anything I could not handle with His help. I simply prayed over and over for God's will to be done and for me to have the strength, the courage, and the willingness to accept whatever it might be, as well as to be there for my parents. I went to lots of meetings, shared and cried, and my Higher Power and the C.A. Fellowship carried me. My father died just three weeks later, and although losing him was the worst experience in my life, I never once wanted to drink or use. It wasn't easy, but I made it through his death sober, one day at a time. I know now that there's nothing worth using or drinking over.

I can't say enough about what the C.A. Fellowship has done for me. I finally feel "a part of" instead of "apart from." The first C.A. meeting I went to has been my home group ever since. I've made better friends in C.A. than I ever thought I'd have—or deserved. They have loved and supported me through the few really bad times I've had in sobriety and have been there for the many, many good times.

Working the Steps has changed my life for the better in so many ways. I thought I would always want to get high but would somehow learn to control it. I was delighted to realize, somewhere between Steps Five and Nine, that the urges and cravings had gone away. What a miracle!

Today I know what it is to be happy, joyous, and free. In so many ways, I am a vastly different person than when I got here. Instead of being homeless, unemployable, and destitute, I own my home, have a good job, drive a nice car, and have money in the bank, but it's the way I feel inside that's the real miracle. That hole in my soul is gone, hopefully never to return, and I no longer feel alone. The spiritual aspect of this program that I fought so hard in the beginning has become my lifeline. I have absolutely priceless relationships with my friends and family, and with God, and I truly love the person I see in the mirror today. It feels so good to know who I am and to finally be able to be the same person everywhere I go.

I understand today that I could never have achieved this transformation on my own; I needed the help of a Higher Power. The decision I made in Step Three would have meant nothing if I hadn't followed it up by working the rest of the Steps. As long as I do a few simple things on a daily basis, I am blessed with an incredibly good quality of life. In my experience, cutting back on prayer and meditation to save time is always poor economy. The few minutes I spend connecting with my Higher Power each day make every other minute of my day that much better. Nowadays

I'd no sooner leave the house in the morning without praying first than I would without brushing my teeth.

I still go to meetings because I love going to meetings, and because I love carrying the message that this program works. I keep working the Steps because they work, and I've got plenty of growing left to do. I still do service because I want to keep giving back to the Fellowship that saved my life, and because I always want C.A. to be there for people like me. I keep praying because I know I would be totally lost without my Higher Power. I still make a gratitude list every day as my first sponsor suggested, but nowadays it's hard to narrow my gratitude list to only five items. I thank God every morning and every night for a number of things, starting with my relationships with my friends and my family and ending by thanking Him most of all for my recovery because without that, I wouldn't have anything.

I've learned that when I'm experiencing a lack of serenity, it's invariably because I'm not getting my way, and I need to remember to relax because God's in charge. I've learned that when I let Him, God really does do for me what I could not do for myself. I've learned that it really is about the journey, not the destination, and I'm no longer worried about when I'll get "there." With each passing year I understand the program a little better, gain more understanding of who I am and how to be a better person, and grow closer to my Higher Power. I've learned that I'll never be done with my recovery, that it's a lifelong process, and most of all that I still have so much to learn. To be honest, I wouldn't have it any other way. I look forward to each new day of my recovery, and I am forever grateful to Cocaine Anonymous.

14

INSIDE OUT AND BACK AGAIN

He went from the brink of insanity to the leading edge of a beautiful adventure.

When I walked through the doors of recovery, I was completely powerless over drugs and alcohol. They ran my life. Everything I did revolved around surviving in the world of my addictions. If I worked, it was to have more money to use. When I woke up, I would find a way to use until the time I would sleep. I had no choice. I didn't even know that I had no choice, that I was powerless. I did not understand that I was killing myself, and placing myself in situations where I could die.

I lived in the chaos of my own insanity much of my life. The things that I did were not normal to anyone except me. From the outside looking in, my life was a mess. From the inside looking out, I couldn't see it. Even if people tried to tell me how screwed up I was, I couldn't understand. I would think that they were square. They could not possibly feel the loneliness or discontentment that I felt. They could not understand how my head reeled with what seemed like a thousand thoughts in a second. They could not understand how I would wake up every day in a state of fear that paralyzed me. I had no idea that living in constant fear was not normal. I did not understand that I was different, that a void existed in me that I could not fill.

What I did know was that when I used—when I drank, smoked, snorted, or popped a hit of acid—things changed. My life became at least bearable. When I was high, those feelings of uselessness, despair, self-pity, and fear were no longer as prevalent. I didn't know that the internal workings of my diseased mind would continue to drive me further and further down the path of self-destruction, self-hatred, and insanity. Over the years I grew steadily more and more dependent on something that was no longer working. I never realized the fog that created the world that I lived in was drug-induced. The more I used, the denser the fog became, until something snapped.

I cannot name a date, time, or location for when the change occurred, I can only say that those things that once worked for me began to fail. Using, which had been my answer, no longer quieted that internal feeling of discontent, fear, anger, and resentment. I no longer had any control over any aspect of my life. What once soothed me was now intensifying everything inside of me that it used to calm. I finally hit my bottom. I was totally devoid of all reason. I was spiritually and mentally bankrupt, a shell of a man consumed by his disease.

What happened next was unexplainable—completely contrary to all that I believed at the time. I have heard it explained as a moment of clarity. It was at the end of a four-day binge that had started on a Thursday with one drink, followed by the thought of one quarter gram, followed by sitting down at the glass table of one of the seven dealers I was distributing for at the time. On Friday I called in sick at my regular job. Saturday night I was still sitting in the same seat around that glass table. After two days, I finally got out of that seat and cleaned up. That night, the dealer and I headed out for the bars. By midnight we were set up in one of the local taverns.

There was nothing about this behavior that had not been acted out many times before, nothing extraordinary about that night, or about anything that led to the following thought. The words just flowed out of my mouth. I turned to my dealer and said, "I have to stop. This is getting crazy." He agreed, and for a short time after, we discussed how we would do this together at his house the next weekend.

But I knew as soon as the conversation began that there was no way we could accomplish that goal together. By this point in my using career, I had tried several ways of quitting: cold turkey, switching addictions, and geographical escapes. None of them worked. I knew that I was not capable of quitting, let alone quitting with one of my drug dealers. Sunday rolled around, and we found ourselves sitting in another bar. The drugs were all gone, and the beers were swishing down my throat, yet the idea of quitting was still fresh in my mind. At noon I sloshed down that last gulp of beer. My glass hit the bar, and the bartender reached for it. I quickly put my hand over the top and said, "I'm done. I am going home."

The second part of the miracle happened the next day. I was at work, in a state of shock and confusion. I was holding an electrical component that I was to repair, a job I had done a thousand times before, something that had become second nature to me. Yet there I was, motionless, alone, confused, and in a moment of consuming fear. I had no clue what to do next. My mind was racing so fast, creating scenarios of the night before, the night after, what I should do next time, what I should have done, where I would go, who I would see, who I had seen, how I would get high, how I would pay for it all. I could not stop the incessant rambling inside my head. I could not figure out, through all of this noise, what to do next. I was paralyzed in fear.

I knew I needed help. I walked away from that job and into my boss' office, where I declared that I was going to sign myself into a local treatment center that night. He turned to me and said very simply, "I think that is a good idea. Don't worry about anything on this end, I will handle it."

I don't remember the rest of that day, until arriving at my parents' house that evening. I was 29 years old and living under their roof. I was not capable of any other life. My father was sober for three years by this time. I really knew nothing about his recovery, considering I had been in this overwhelming fog for much longer than that, but I did remember he entered treatment for help. So there I was, pacing inside the house when he walked in. I mentioned to him that I wanted to go to treatment. The next thing I knew he was on the phone and asking me questions. I found out later that the facility was going to put off my coming in until the next day, but he would not have any of that. He convinced them that the situation was critical and got off the phone saying they were ready for me.

Fear set in, and I said, "I have to watch my favorite TV show first." Reluctantly he agreed. I went up to my little room on the second floor and turned on the TV. Not more than a minute later, I was trying to figure out how to get out of that house without being caught. I was about to head for the second-story window so I could jump when my dad walked through the door saying he thought we should leave now. I just do not argue with my dad, so I got into his car, and we headed for the treatment center.

On the way I mentioned how maybe we should stop for a beer. His response was "I don't think that's a good idea, do you?" My head screamed, "*Yes!*" but my mouth said, "No."

Fear gripped me as we walked through the glass doors of a brick treatment center that looked to me like a prison. I was afraid of living, I was afraid of dying, I was afraid of using, I was afraid of staying clean. But I found myself answering all the questions presented to me at the time with as much honesty as I could muster.

I was checked in for 28 days. They secluded me from all my outside distractions. On the third day I remember looking out the window. It was Halloween, a big party night. I started pacing between the window and the locker, which held my coat. Back and forth I paced. My mind raced. All I could think was, "I cannot do this. I cannot face this world sober."

Then something happened. I looked out the window again. It was fall, and for the first time for as far back as I could remember, I saw color—bright, wonderful color. I was immediately overwhelmed.

Today I can see how God's grace kept me there that night. While I was in treatment, I was introduced to Cocaine Anonymous. I started to find some answers from the very first hug at the door of that very first meeting, and I can remember calling myself an addict for the very first time. I can remember the freedom behind speaking those words. I knew the answer for me lay within those walls, and yet I had no clue what that answer was.

The night I was released, I found myself driving around the block of my favorite tavern. Around and around I went, searching for a way to stop the insanity in my head. My disease was rampant. I finally walked into the bar, and my head quieted. I did not drink, yet the cunning, baffling, and powerful nature of my disease took over. At first it was just making me comfortable with being around using people. Next it told me I should drink a nonalcoholic beer to fit in.

I was going to meetings, spewing what I believed to be the recovery program out of my mouth, but there was no substance behind my words. I picked a sponsor who never made me work, and I went to meetings because I liked the girls. Within four months I found myself in a dangerous place. At a friend's house one night, a familiar aroma made me forget everything that brought me into recovery to begin with. When I searched out the source of the smell, I found my friend hitting off the pipe, and I asked for a hit. He refused, but I convinced him that just one wouldn't hurt.

Two weeks later I found myself surrounded by the same insanity and mental condition as the first day I walked through the doors of the treatment center. I walked into a meeting completely whooped again. When I told my sponsor of my relapse, he asked me to turn around. I did. He asked me to bend over. I did. Then he literally kicked me in the ass and said, "Okay, now it's time to work."

That night I stood up at a meeting of about one hundred people and told my story. Then I asked for their help, and we broke off into groups. I might have heard the first person talk before my disease took control. My mind raced, and I was overwhelmed with the desire to leave and find the dope that I had stashed at my friend's house. Thank God for my massive ego at the time. After my grandiose display of asking for help, I knew I could not just get up and leave. When the meeting ended, I bolted for the door, trying to avoid my sponsor. He caught me and asked how I felt. I answered, "I feel like using." He said, "Good." I wanted to punch him, but we talked, and I went home that night thinking about what he had said. God's grace had intervened.

So began my incredible journey of recovery. My sponsor started talking to me about God, but I was not willing to hear anything he said—until the next craving set in. On an evening filled with fear and desperation, he explained to me how spirituality and religion are different. He suggested that I walk out my back door and ask for help. He explained to me that I did not have to know who I was asking help from, I just had to do it.

I had no other choice, so I tried it. It worked. I blew it off as coincidence, but I had a reasonable doubt, so I tried again, and it worked again. I blew it off again. I did not want to believe, but I kept trying this suggestion, and it kept working until I had no other choice but to believe. I began to understand God as something of great importance in my life. I began to have faith that with God I can walk through my fears. I began to understand that if I would direct my life onto the path that He prescribed for me, wonderful things would come to pass.

My sponsor guided me through Steps Four through Seven. I walked in faith despite my fears, and I began to change. I began to see how the defects that once helped me survive were now destroying my chances. With my sponsor's help, I set out to clean up my past through the Eighth and Ninth Steps. I began to feel certain freedoms and to see the Promises come true.

Many of these lessons of recovery were hard-fought. For a long time I rode a roller coaster of emotions, and yet I found that I could walk through them with a clear, uncluttered mind. To be able to think that clearly and precisely, to have only one thought rather than a hundred raging voices, is one of the greatest gifts recovery handed me.

When I do make mistakes, working the Tenth Step affords me the opportunity to clean them up right away and to keep my clarity of mind. The Eleventh Step has allowed me to stay open to the direction of the will of God (as I understand Him), on a minute-to-minute basis. I can check myself every night, review my day, and ensure I stay on a spiritual path. When I awake in the morning, I ask for the strength to carry out His will throughout my day. The Eleventh Step coupled with the Tenth allows me to stay grounded in the moment and out of the way of myself.

I have been handed this great gift from God and the Fellowship, an exciting new life full of unlimited adventure and discovery. That's a debt that no matter how hard I try, I will never have the ability to repay. One of the most wonderful parts of recovery is to watch a fellow addict evolve in the spirit, to watch as someone's lights go on for the very first time, recognizing that a Higher Power is there. I have held men in my arms, both of us crying from relief, as they have passed from that place of despair and desperation into the world of hope. I have seen how they struggle through the Steps to walk out a whole individual full of strength and character. I have seen how they have embraced this gift and flourished and become one of God's unbelievable works of art.

I am a fallible human being with a disease that is cunning, baffling, and powerful. I do not have the capability of working this program perfectly, and in the past 12 years I have on occasion found myself amidst personal chaos. There have even been times where I have not been able to recognize that I am in a state of personal insanity. When I start to feel that clear thinking fade or recognize that it is gone completely, I know something in my life is wrong.

Sometimes these situations were brought about by my lack of working the program to the best of my ability. The solution for this has been as simple as beginning to pray again in the morning, keeping an open communication between God and myself, going to more meetings, working harder with others, and becoming more involved with service work. Other times it becomes more complicated than that. I could be doing everything the program asks of me and still feel uncomfortable in my life. These are times of evolution for me. These times have afforded me the opportunity to restart and relive this wonderful adventure all over again. There are times life takes me back to powerlessness and unmanageability. There are times life allows me to reconnect with God. There are times life forces me back into the Fifth through the Ninth Steps. At all of these times, I continue to grow.

Every time I walk through the Steps of this program, I learn to better understand my place in God's world. Every time I pick up the "Big Book" or the "Twelve and Twelve," I see new things that I have never seen before. Each time this happens I become inspired again, full of new life and enthusiasm to leap forward onto a new plane of spiritual existence. The great part of it all is that it never ends. As many times as I have thought I reached the ultimate plateau, I have found that there is one even greater. I know extremely little of the wonderful gifts this life and this adventure have to offer me. I am a living, breathing example that the recovery program of Cocaine Anonymous works.

When I walked into this Fellowship 12 years ago, it was fairly new in this area, and to see someone with five years of sobriety was a bit of a novelty. I have watched as this Fellowship of C.A. grew from its struggles of infancy into a thriving force of lifesaving grace. Like my personal program of recovery, I can see how we as a Fellowship are evolving. Even at the meeting level, I can see how things are changing and progressing.

Sometimes I get choked up with gratitude as I look around and see the faces of those I have grown up with in these rooms. I respect and admire these people. I know where they came from and how hard they had to work to beat the odds. They share their experience, strength, and hope with newcomers and old-timers alike. They never deserted the Fellowship that saved their lives. They fought and clawed their way through a lot of adversity to come out shining stars.

15

A LIAR, A CHEAT, A THIEF AND A WHORE

She went from the bottom of her addiction to being a proud and grateful member of Cocaine Anonymous.

I came to in a dark, cold, rubber room. I was naked except for a little blue paper gown. Suddenly I was struck with the memory of what had happened, where I'd been, and how I'd come to end up in this stinky brown hell. I remembered being handcuffed to a bench in a holding cell. I was crying and screaming at my husband, who was in the cell next to me, and I was banging my wrists against the handcuffs. I thought I might break free any second. I remembered having my picture taken and being fingerprinted. I remembered being arrested on my grandmother's front porch. Oh, and that look on her face—how could I forget the look of horror, of despair, of total shock and disappointment? She didn't want to believe that I had broken into her store and stolen $40 out of the register. She didn't want to believe that I had set off the alarm and sat before her lying when the alarm company called. She didn't want to believe it was me, but somehow she knew it was. I'll never forget her face, her sad, sad eyes.

The destruction that followed that spree was the worst of all my sprees—and that time I got caught. My mother bailed my husband and me out of jail for the last time. My entire family was dragged into court to testify as to whether or not I was authorized to be in the store that night. My uncle was partial owner of the store, and he was not going to let me get away with this one. Because of my selfishness, my self-centeredness, because of my addiction to crack cocaine, my entire family was falling apart before my very eyes. A moment of clarity struck me, and I went to my public defender and asked for a break, a plea bargain, anything to avoid having my 77-year-old grandmother testify in court. The public defender asked if I was willing to go to rehab. Of course I was. Rehab sounded like a vacation to me. Once I got there, it took me quite a long time to discover that I might have a problem.

I thought maybe rehab would teach me how to only smoke crack on Fridays or maybe just once a month, or how to take one or two hits and walk away from the pipe. That's still the funniest thing I've ever heard myself say. I definitely didn't think I had a drinking problem, and I wasn't going to admit to the other drugs I had been doing most of my life. Crack was what made me break into that store. Crack was what landed me in the padded cell in county jail. Crack was what I was in rehab for. That's it. Nothing more. Just crack. And I wasn't going to call myself an addict or alcoholic because I never used needles or drank out of brown paper bags.

When I got out of rehab, I was faced with life again. What a terrifying feeling. I felt like I imagine a burn victim would feel: raw, unprotected, sore, itchy, ashamed, afraid, and alone. I was afraid to leave my house, but I was afraid to stay home. I was afraid to ask for help, but I was afraid not to. I was afraid of everything and nothing, everyone and no one. And the worst part of all of it was that I didn't even know who I was or who I wanted to be. I didn't know where to begin, but I knew something had to change. I prayed for something or someone to help me.

I had somehow accumulated 27 consecutive days clean and sober when my husband and I went to a party at a bar. All of my husband's coworkers were there, and everyone was drinking. We ordered coffee and drank pot after pot. One of the servers accidentally set a shot of tequila down in front of me. It had happened once earlier with another server, but this time was different. Before I even thought about it, the tequila was going down my throat to my stomach, and before my shot glass hit the table I had ordered another one. By the time the second shot was in my belly, I knew I was in trouble. I felt my toes get tingly, and then the feeling crept slowly up my legs, into my stomach and chest, until my head was tingly. I knew in the pit of my stomach that something terrible was about to happen.

I grabbed my husband and tried to drag him out the door. He had seen me take the shots and had ordered two for himself. He didn't want to go, he wanted to stay and have more. I finally convinced him to come with me. The entire ride home we fought about whether or not to stop and buy some beer. Before I knew it, we were in the driveway of our house. Somehow we'd gotten home without buying more alcohol. I was relieved, but a little irritated. A huge part of me wanted to get some beer, but a bigger part of me knew what would follow a few beers: a trip to the dealer's house; home to do all the dope in five minutes or less; another trip to the dealer's house; another trip home. Somewhere in all that we would have to find more money for dope, and I didn't want to go back to that rubber room ever again. I went inside and went to bed.

When I woke up the next morning, I wasn't hung over, I wasn't sick at all, and I had slept hard the entire night. I knew that something had happened in my life. I knew that the prayer I had prayed a few weeks prior had been answered. Something had helped me. Something got me home from the bar the night before, and that something kept me from getting high again. I was excited to make it to a meeting and share my experience with everyone else. I was excited to recommit myself. I was excited because I knew somehow everything was going to be all right. Somehow, some way, I could make it, clean and sober with a little help from my newfound sober friends.

I got my hands on a Step Guide. I thought I would have it all figured out on my own in no time. I started answering the questions in the guide like they were homework and I would be graded on my answers. I called a lady about once a week and asked her to listen to my answers. She showed up twice and listened to me. She didn't say much, but she would always offer some of her own experiences for contrast. After the second time, she was always too busy to meet me, so I continued working on my own. I got about two pages into the Fourth Step and started feeling absolutely insane. I quit the Step work altogether. I stayed sick and miserable for a few more months.

There was another woman who was close to my age whom I had seen at some meetings. She seemed so fun, free, passionate, and clean and sober. I was always attracted to her when she spoke, and I wanted what she had. She had given me her phone number at a meeting once, but I had never used it. I was scared to. What if she didn't like me? I thought for sure that if I told her anything about me, about what I had done, she would hate me. I wanted her to be my sponsor, but I didn't ask her because I was afraid of what she would say. If she said yes, I would have to share myself with her. If she said no, it would be another rejection, and I couldn't take any more rejections.

Eight days after my first clean and sober birthday, I asked her to sponsor me. She asked me if I had a problem with God. I said, "No problems. I'm willing to believe today." She agreed to be my sponsor and hugged me. I will never forget that moment. I knew deep down inside that she had what I wanted and needed to save my own life.

She told me to call her every day, go to a meeting every day, and she gave me a reading assignment. She said to tell her when I finished the assignment, and she would tell me how she wrote out her First Step. I read it that night and called her the next day. She took me through the Steps, one by one. When we got to my Third Step, she asked me how I prayed. I told her I would usually just say whatever was on my mind when I went to bed. My sponsor shared with me how to ask God for guidance throughout the day and how to thank God for my day before going to bed. When she got on her knees and prayed the Third Step Prayer with me, I felt a lightning bolt inside of me. I felt freedom for the first time in a long time. I had arrived.

I wrote out a Fourth Step. I wrote some outrageous things, about how everyone else had hurt me, lied to me, stolen from me. When I got to my sponsor's house to go over it with her and give her my Fifth Step, she said it was time for the fourth column. I'd read nothing about a fourth column and assured her that she must be crazy. She said it was time for me to write down my part in every one of those resentments and fears. My part? I had none. Those people had hurt me. She said we wouldn't be leaving her bedroom until I was finished. I wanted to stab her with my pencil, but instead I started looking inside of me and writing about it. What a freeing feeling it was to tell her that I was a liar, a cheat, a thief and a whore. What a relief it was to no longer hold such anger, hate, shame and guilt inside of me.

There were some terrible things on those pages of my Fourth Step by the time I finished with it. During the process of my Fifth Step, sharing my experiences as a liar, a cheat, a thief and a whore, my sponsor cried with me. She laughed with me. She hugged me and told me she loved me. She listened, and when I finished she shared some things with me that she had done. The most important things that she did for me were to love me, hug me and tell me that I never had to do any of those things again. I never had to feel that way again. That night I slept like a baby, as I have just about every night since.

Through the process of working the Steps, admitting my wrongs, seeing the error in my ways, making amends where due, and helping other people like me, I found the me that I never knew existed. I also found a loving, forgiving God, some very dear friends, and freedom from a hopeless state of mind and body. I have learned how to work the Steps in my life every day. I have learned how to apply the Twelve Traditions to my personal life and my relationships. I have learned to stay teachable. I have become involved in service to Cocaine Anonymous and have learned responsibility, trust, and unity. It is a privilege and an honor to be a part of C.A. and to watch this Fellowship grow and carry the message to sick and suffering addicts and alcoholics. Cocaine Anonymous opened its arms to me and gave me a safe place to be me. Today I am a proud and grateful member of Cocaine Anonymous, and God willing, in eight days, this alcoholic and addict will celebrate three years clean and sober. I am forever grateful to this program for showing me the way.

16

OUT OF DESTRUCTION AND FEAR

He lied, cheated and stole his way to the bottom until his sister carried the message that led him to recovery.

I come from a middle-class home in the suburbs of a large American city. I am the third of four children, with two older sisters and a younger brother. I was born a very curious and needful person. I can remember always wanting more—more attention, more toys, more friends. My addictive behavior started at a very early age. It didn't seem to matter what it was; if I thought I liked it, I wanted more.

Our family moved from the Northeast to the Southwest when I was 10 years old. My life changed drastically, and I felt I had lost control of everything. My father was a hardworking man with good values who tried his best to provide for his family. When we moved, I felt I lost my father's attention. It was because he was working multiple jobs to support us, but I didn't see that; all I saw was that I wasn't spending the time with him that I was accustomed to. It seemed the only attention I got from him was when I did something wrong, and he would have to sit me down and talk to me about my bad behavior. Needless to say, my behavior got worse, not better.

Soon after we moved, I had my first beer with some of my sister's friends. I really didn't care for the taste, but I did like the attention I got from these older guys. I didn't have just one, I drank until I was puking. I got home very late and continued to puke some more.

My father accused me of being on drugs and sent me to bed. When I woke up the next day, my mother asked me what I had been doing the night before, and I told her I was drinking. She told me that I should learn a lesson from this and left it at that.

I remember that all I could think about was how I could repeat the events of the previous night. I did not like the taste of the beer; I did not like to puke my guts out. What I did like was the attention I got from my sister's boyfriends and the fact that my father didn't like what I was doing. I had come to the conclusion that if my father didn't want to be with me, I would do the exact opposite of what he wanted me to do, no matter what it was.

At the age of 14, I came to another conclusion—that I had all the answers to be had around there, and that to get more answers, I would need to travel the world. A friend and I stole one of my father's company cars and made it about 80 miles east of the metro area. When the car ran out of gas, my friend decided he'd had enough fun and went home. I was sure that I had nothing to go back for, so I continued on my journey to conquer the world.

As my drinking got heavier, my behavior got worse. I got more violent as time went on. I was the guy who would see someone with something I wanted, get in his or her face and take it, hoping for an argument. This behavior got me locked up in a variety of institutions. By the time I was 19, I had spent half of the previous nine years locked up in one institution or another. Jails and hospitals had become a safe haven for me, a place to sober up, eat, and catch up on my rest.

My probation officer told me that if I violated probation one more time, I was going to prison. I didn't care for the thought of prison, so I came up with a plan to fix my problem. I concluded that I was probably an alcoholic and that I needed to get away from those around me who were causing me to continue down this path of ruin. It never entered my mind that by taking off again I was violating my probation.

I hit the road and ended up on the southern Atlantic coast a week later, without any alcohol in my system and feeling like one very large raw nerve exposed to the world. I was a little afraid of drugs but was willing to try anything that could possibly be considered fun. I bought a physician's reference guide for prescription drugs so that I could read about any drug that came my way and then decide if I should take it or not. I used this guide for about six months.

Never once did I read about a drug and its effects and decide not to take it.

Then my life took a completely different shape. I found that I really liked pot. I enjoyed everything about it—taste, smell, looks, and portability. I was open to trying anything new, and along with the pot were a wide variety of other drugs that came in all sizes, shapes, and forms. I noticed that I was no longer acting violent. I much preferred to kick back and watch than get into any kind of confrontation. If you had something I wanted I would sneak around behind your back and take it when you weren't looking. Then when you realized it was missing, I would help you look for it. This behavior seemed to be working for me very well. I was no longer ending up in jails or hospitals.

I decided that I had changed my life from bad to positive because I hadn't gotten locked up for two years. Now I could go back home and show my probation officer what a good person I had become.

In order to fulfill my dreams, I needed to get rich and famous. I enrolled in a school for broadcasting. I wanted to become a disc jockey so all the world would love me. I excelled in my classes and was employed before I graduated. I thought I had the world in the palm of my hand.

My drug use progressed to the point where I would spend days at a time locked in the radio station production studio perfecting my craft. A couple of years into my new career, the station I was working for hired a new general manager. I was sure that this meant I would lose my job, so I quit before he could fire me. I was sure that every nearby station would want me. I was wrong. I spent the next six months looking for work, spiraling downward like an airplane out of control. Emotionally, mentally, and physically I was going down.

I came to the conclusion that I needed to move to a smaller radio market. Instead of being the on-air/production staff, I decided that I needed to be the manager of the entire station. Amazingly, I got a job as the programming/production manager of a station in a small town. This fit into my plan well because by this time I also realized that I had a drug problem, and I believed that by moving I could get away from all my bad influences. I made it about three months without any drugs or alcohol.

One night after work, I joined a coworker at a pool hall. He bought a pitcher of beer. Being a nice guy, he offered me some. My first reaction was to say no. I had trained myself to say no to alcohol. Then I thought about it. My mind said to me, "You haven't had a beer in 10 years. You have a drug problem now, not a drinking problem." I had one beer that night. It sent me off on a binge that I never could have imagined. I managed to destroy everything in my path for the next two years, drinking and doing drugs at rates that I could not control.

I ended up in a total state of confusion. I had never felt so bad in my life. Nothing seemed to work for me. I had lied, cheated, and stolen my way to the bottom. I felt worse than ever about myself. I lost every bit of hope I ever had. I considered killing myself but couldn't bring myself to do it. I loaded up my truck with everything I could fit in it, including a large amount of pot. I then took off looking for the answers to my problems, not knowing what my problems were.

The only thing I knew for sure was that I was tired of hurting people. It seemed that everyone I came into contact with, I hurt physically, mentally, or emotionally. I ended up in a church. I spent the next hour or so telling the preacher everything I had done. After I finished, he looked at me and told me I definitely had a problem but that he couldn't help me. I was lost. I went back to my hotel room and hit my knees, crying, praying for help. I just wanted to stop feeling so lost, helpless, and out of control.

The next day found me on the road again and full of fear that I could very well end up dead, or worse. I told myself on the way that I was not going to ask anyone I knew for any help, for fear that I would hurt them again.

When I reached my hometown, I called my mother, not knowing who else to call. When she answered the phone and realized who it was, I could hear the fear in her voice. I didn't know how my own mother could be afraid of me. I asked if I could come see her, and reluctantly she agreed. I arrived at her home scared to death of what could happen. The mutual fear was too much for me to take. She and my grandmother were afraid of me, and I couldn't understand why. This scared me, and I wanted to run. I asked my mother for my sisters' and brother's phone numbers. She said she wouldn't do that to them, but that if I left my phone number, she would give it to them.

A couple of days later my older sister called me. She asked me how I was. I told her everything was great and that I was back to take on the world. She laughed. I asked her how she was, and she replied that she was okay. I asked if we could get together to catch up and talk. She said that sounded good and that she and her roommate were going to a meeting that night, followed by a dance, and I was welcome to come.

The last time I had seen my sister she had checked herself into a detox ward at a hospital to take care of her drinking problem. I had never been to a meeting, but I had an idea what she was talking about. Some of my friends had to go to meetings because of their troubles with the law. I didn't understand why my sister still went to meetings, since I assumed she had gotten "cured" in detox. But I wanted to see her, so I agreed.

They picked me up, and we went to a Twelve-Step meeting where one of her sponsees was sharing. I walked into the room, and to my surprise, everyone treated me like I was a lost friend. They were all very happy to see me, hugging me and welcoming me to the meeting. I was stunned.

Then the meeting started. Here was a girl 10 years younger than me telling everyone in the room everything I had ever done. To me it sounded as if she was sharing with everyone how I felt about myself and all of the terrible things I had done to people over the years. I was confused and couldn't figure out how this girl knew me so well. How dare she tell on me? I was going through my two emotions (angry and happy) like a tornado. I left that meeting with a lot of questions.

On the way to the dance, I sat in the back seat of the car, listening to my sister and her roommate talk, not really hearing what was said. I was too busy in my own head trying to figure out how I had gotten to this point and what to do about it.

We got to the dance, and again I couldn't believe what was happening. I was greeted like a long-lost friend by a bunch of complete strangers, hugging me and acting truly happy to see me. I had never experienced this kind of attention before. These were people from all different walks of life. As I looked around the room, I was amazed at how two or three hundred people who obviously should not belong together could be having so much fun, especially when they all claimed to be clean and sober.

After the dance we left, and all I could think of was how I could be part of this thing. How could I be happy like they all seemed to be? I asked my sister and her roommate what was going on and what I needed to do to be part of it. All they would tell me was that I needed to get a sponsor and do whatever he told me to do. Then they handed me a meeting list and said I needed to go to meetings every day. At this point I was willing to try anything; after all, it wasn't like I had anything else to do. I could see my sister looking happier than I had ever seen her, with a lot of friends and a life.

As it turned out, she had managed to stay sober for over five years by being part of this program called Cocaine Anonymous. I had one more night in my hotel room with no money, no job, and only the hope that C.A. might help. I spent the next few days going to meetings, then to coffee afterward, trying to see what this C.A. thing was all about. After coffee, I would go to the park closest to the meeting and spend the night. I seemed to run into my sister at every meeting, and it looked like everyone in the meetings knew her and liked her. I was even more curious, but not sure it would work for me.

One night after a meeting, my sister came up to me and asked if I had gotten a sponsor yet. I really wanted to lie and say I had, but for the first time in my life, I thought about it. I thought if I told her I did, she would ask who, I'd give her a name, and she would find out I was lying. So I told her no. She grabbed me, introduced me to a guy, and said he would make a great sponsor. I looked at him, knowing from all the meetings I had attended what was supposed to happen next. I asked him if he would be my sponsor. He replied, "Are you willing to go to any lengths to stay clean and sober?" I knew what he wanted to hear, so I said yes. He asked me to call him every day. I said I was broke and didn't have a phone. He reached into his pocket and handed me $10 and said, "Will you call me every day?" I reluctantly said yes.

I knew that if I got a sponsor, I would be expected to do what he told me to do, and I am not the kind of person who does what others tell me to do very well. I am more apt to do the opposite. However, something came over me. I thought, "I'll try this thing the way they tell me to do it, and when it doesn't work, I'll be able to blame them for all my problems."

The next day I called my sponsor, and we talked for a long while about how I had come to this point in my life. He left me with a reading assignment and told me to call him every day in the meantime. I had nothing else to do. The next meeting wasn't until later that night, so I sat in my car and started reading. I took a break to go to the meeting and coffee. Then I went to the park and finished the assignment my sponsor had given me. I called him in the morning, and he said it was time to start working the Steps.

I had no problem admitting that I was an addict and that my life was unmanageable; I was living in my car in the park closest to the last meeting I attended. And I certainly had no control over anything in my life. I had proven to myself that no human power could relieve the pain I was feeling.

As far as believing in a Power greater than myself, I knew that God existed; I was also sure that He wanted nothing to do with me.

My sponsor said that I needed to change my perception of God. He told me to write a list of all the characteristics I wanted in a best friend and to have it ready the next day. When we met at the meeting that night, we went over my list, and he wrote at the top of it "My Higher Power" and told me I needed to turn my will and my life over to my Higher Power. He told me the way to do that was to start praying for the strength to stay clean and sober every morning and to thank Him every night. He then said I needed to start on my Fourth Step, writing a list of everyone I resented or had harmed.

We got together the next day and went over my list, reviewing the cause of the resentment, how it affected me, and what my part in the resentment was. I was seeing just how full of fear I was and how fear had the power to make me do all kinds of things. I came to realize that I was an egomaniac with an inferiority complex. Next we reviewed my past relationships. He showed me where I was selfish and self-centered. Then he told me to go home and sit quietly, reviewing what we had just done, and pray for guidance to see if I'd left anything out.

For the next couple hours, I was in a state of overwhelming relief and accomplishment. For the first time in my life, I felt like I could actually do anything I wanted to do. I began to pray to God for the strength, the courage, and the willingness to do His will.

The next day I called my sponsor, and he told me I needed to start using the Third and Seventh Step Prayers on a daily basis, and that it was time to start making amends to those I had harmed. I started with my family and worked my way down the list. I've had many different responses, from people being very happy that I've become a useful person in society to others who didn't want to hear it. What I've learned is that as long as I'm willing, God will take care of the results.

My sponsor also told me I needed to review my day before bed every night and start the process of taking care of my resentments as they happen instead of storing them up and exploding. I also had to correct any bad behavior on my part as soon as possible.

My sponsor then led me into being of service. It started with getting to meetings early and helping set up, then staying late and cleaning up before going to coffee. In the beginning, I didn't understand the need for this. As time went on, I came to realize that it is these types of actions that rebuild my self-esteem. I was taken to our H&I Committee meeting where I was assigned to chair a meeting in a halfway house that catered to the federal prison system. What an experience that was: I got to see firsthand the power of fear in others' lives, and how denial can drive a person to drink and use drugs. My first service commitment came from the H&I Committee as well. I was the co-chair for the H&I Chips and Literature Committee—talk about work! This position showed me the importance of an inventory and how valuable a tool it can be in all areas of my life.

Then came my first sponsee. I got the opportunity to guide another person through the Steps. What an incredible learning experience. I don't know if I was of any help to him, but being a sponsor helped me learn more about myself than anything else I'd done. I can go on and on about how I feel when it comes to C.A. and the opportunities this program has given me. I believe that a person has to be of service in life in order to feel a part of society. Since I've been in the program, I have come a long way from being a fear-driven person who merely reacts to situations.

Today I don't have the need to be surrounded by large amounts of chaos. I'm much more comfortable doing things the right way and not having to go through the consequences of my bad behavior. I've also had the opportunity to realize what my dreams are, and, by the grace of God, I have fulfilled a few. I live life to the best of my ability by going out and doing things I always talked about someday doing when I was using. I try anything new that comes my way, whether it's a new cuisine or going to a ball game (I'm not a sports fan).

I have a great, active relationship with my family now. Since my father died, they look to me for guidance and direction. What a trip!

I got engaged this year to a wonderful woman. She has a great family, and her father and his wife gave us a trip overseas. That's incredible. What's even more incredible is that we get to go with them. Let me emphasize this: we get to go with them. Not only am I in the position to take off work, I can afford to take off work and hang out abroad with my future in-laws. In the past, nobody would have taken me to a fast food restaurant, much less another country.

My father always told me that I'd be lucky to have one good friend who I could count on to tell me the truth no matter what it was, to hold me when times were tough, and to play with when times were good. Today I have more of these friends than I could ever spend time with. These people are the ones who refer to me as dependable, stable, kind, and loving. They say I have things like integrity and charisma. People treat me with respect and kindness, and I am blown away.

17

FROM DOMINANCE TO SURRENDER

Finding a Higher Power of her own understanding allowed her to become a free and happy woman.

Before I got sober, I thought I was the greatest power in my part of the world. Many men would have agreed with me because it was my job to make them believe that. Being a dominatrix was a perfect job for me because I was a woman who needed to do a lot of cocaine and wanted to hit people. But the fact is that as I write this story, it's been over four thousand days since I last smoked any cocaine. That's meaningful to me.

When I was young, I figured out that I could get what I wanted by manipulating other people through what I said, what I wore, and what I bought them. In fifth grade, I started by hanging out with people who smoked pot. At 13, I was smoking pot and taking bennies and reds. I met a guy who hung out at one of the cemeteries. He shot us up with LSD under our tongues and led us through cool visions. By 17, I was into cocaine. The first time someone gave me a line, I bought the rest of the cocaine she had, which was a gram. Soon after that, the minimum of all purchases was an eight ball. I bought my first kilo with the idea that I could help my friends buy some, but they never quite got over to my house in time. By the time they got there, it was already half gone.

By 17, I had also become an experienced sexual predator. I had learned by then that if I walked up to someone and said, "Do you want to get high?" they would probably have sex with me. One day I met a beautiful, sexy, blonde woman on the beach. She came with me up to my apartment, and we got high. When my roommate got home, I tied him up and did my whole dominance scene. The woman told me she was a slave girl and that I could make a fortune working dominance.

She was right. I began working in the world of S&M and progressed to owning my own clubs.

I was so angry and full of rage. Cocaine was the only thing that could make me feel better. It numbed me and fixed me for a moment. That worked for about 15 years. Then I got so sick of not being able to resist cocaine that I gave up being a dominatrix, and I bought a fishing resort up north.

I went there thinking that if I just could get away from cocaine, I would be fine. I thought I was safe, until I met a very beautiful girl who wanted some cocaine. I did what I always did if a potential sex partner wanted drugs—I found a way to get the drugs, and I started getting her high.

After a couple of weeks, I was angry with myself and in despair. I realized it didn't matter where I went, I was still going to do the same behavior. I decided I had to stop.

So, I went home. On the way, I finished what was in my pipe and dropped it in the trash at a rest stop. I had driven for over two hours when I realized there was one more hit in that pipe. I turned the car around and drove all the way back to get that pipe out of the trash can so I could get one more high. Just one more high. That's what life was about for me.

When I got home, I wanted to die. I thought death would be better than the hell I was living in with the cocaine. I met some people who suggested that I go into a mental ward. I was hospitalized and put on a hold in a lock-down unit. They said I did not really want to kill myself or want to be dead; what I wanted was relief from my pain.

Then they sent me to a Cocaine Anonymous meeting. Someone in the meeting had 18 months free from cocaine. Eighteen months was a long time, in my personal opinion. They sent me back from the meeting with literature that said I didn't have to do this alone and that they would teach me how to do it—by going to meetings, talking to members on the phone, and doing the Steps. So, I started to go to meetings.

I went through 52 sponsors in the first year because I would tell them to go to hell on a weekly basis. They would usually say, "You don't need to call me anymore." I thought, "Great, I didn't want to call you in the first place."

Then I started to do the Steps to the best of my ability. After a while, I understood, finally, that I had no power over cocaine. That was the First Step; I surrendered to that. I had a little trouble with the Second Step—"Came to believe that a Power greater than ourselves could restore us to sanity"—because I had never achieved sanity in my whole life. How could anything restore me to sanity? I was told it meant not getting high. That was all the sanity I could expect, and that was enough for me.

One Saturday a friend of mine came up to my house to help me with my Third Step. He was a homeless guy I fed after the meeting because he had no money. Using food to get him to stick around and talk to me was still manipulation, but I needed help.

I had made a decision to stay sober, but I didn't know how to turn my will and my life over to a Higher Power. My friend told me that it didn't matter what I prayed to, I could pray to anything. He reminded me of a member who said we could pray to the ocean or a doorknob. Thinking that praying to a doorknob was the stupidest thing I had ever heard, and being the jokester that I am, I said, "I'm going to pray to one of my toys here." So I did.

Since this was going to be my Higher Power, I picked my favorite sex toy and put it in a clear shoebox, high above me, on the top shelf of a bookcase. I was going to follow directions exactly and prove that the program was faulty. They could not possibly mean that it didn't matter what I prayed to. At the beginning of every day, I said, "God, keep me sober," and asked God to remove my obsession. At the end of every sober day, I thanked my God.

After months of this practice, I could not deny that prayer was working. I was staying sober. The principles were working in spite of me. Taking yet another suggestion from fellow members, I stopped using that object to help me practice prayer, and came to think of the word "God" as an acronym for "Girls Off Drugs."

In my Fourth Step, I found out that I was a rapist. This was no news bulletin to anyone around me, but I hadn't realized it. I found that I was cruel, inconsiderate, and intolerant. I treated everybody as if I really didn't give a crap what they thought, what they felt, or that they were alive. But I had done a Fourth Step and a Fifth Step, and I was changing. I thank the Steps and my sponsors for that. I thank them for getting me through my fears list and the sex part of my inventory, and for suggesting that I make amends, even if I didn't appreciate the result in the moment.

When I was 18 months sober, I went out on a blind date with a very good-looking man. We'd had a nice dinner and came back to my apartment—my favorite part of the date—and he offered me some cocaine. At that moment, for the first time in my life, I asked myself if I wanted to get high. That's when the magic happened, and I thought, "I'll try this path a little longer." Because I'd had a spiritual awakening as a result of working the Steps, I said no to cocaine, which was huge for me, and I kicked him out of my apartment.

Soon after, I took a chip commitment. Usually, the chip person stands up and says in a really friendly way, "Hi, I'm your chip person. Anyone a newcomer?" Then they hand the new person a newcomer chip and hug them. My approach was a little different. I would stand up and say, "I'm your chip person. There'll be no hugs today. Any newcomers?"

Then I saw a guy come in, meeting after meeting, and I watched him change. I wondered if he was going to get to 30 days without using. He got 30 days, and I was excited for him. Then he got 60 days, and I hugged him. The crowd went wild, clapping and everything. They were all in shock that I hugged someone. That occurred because I had gone through my Steps at that point, and I knew how much recovery I had and how much it helped me. It was the first time I thought about another human being. Doing commitments allowed me to get out of my self-centeredness.

In my fourth year, there was a woman in a jail-alternative rehab, in a lock-down unit. She had asked me to be her sponsor, and we had gone through her First Step and Second Step. She called me one afternoon and said a man who had raped her just arrived in the unit, and she was going to go AWOL. I drove over there right away. We wrote out a Fourth Step together about what had happened, what she was feeling, and what her part had been. They had been doing crack out at the railroad tracks. She had put herself in dangerous places with dangerous people. When it got to the rape, she asked me, "What was my part in that?" I told her she didn't have a part in that. That was his part. All she did was put herself in that position. The man bore the responsibility for raping her. She said, "All rapists are monsters."

At that moment, I realized that even though I couldn't make direct amends to the people I had raped because none of them would talk to me, I had the opportunity to make a living amends. I took a big gulp and said, "What do you think of me?" She said, "You're really nice," and she complimented me for helping newcomers. "I'm a rapist," I told her. She said, "No, not you." I was crying, and I said, "Yep, and I'm proof that people can change. If you work the program, and you do your Steps, and you're willing to be open to all these 'coincidences,' and you're willing to make amends, there's a Higher Power here who has a way for you to heal."

She started crying. I put out my arms, and she let me hold her. For the first time since writing down that I was a rapist, I started to feel forgiveness for my actions. It was one of the best feelings. I felt freedom. I received that freedom because I had been working the Steps and making amends.

I realized that if I show up to be of service to someone, even though I'm there to help another addict out of his or her pain, I get an opportunity to learn and heal. Those things are what have created a spiritual change in who I am.

Now when I pray, I get a sense of how I can be of service. If you had told me I would be able to feel God's will, I would never have believed it. Now that I know I can call on my Higher Power to give me strength, insight, and support, it's my duty to do things in service, to ask for support and energy for service. Because when I'm doing that, I feel better, stronger.

One of the things I learned in this program is how to love myself. I was taught to write down all the things that made me happy each day, and the qualities, talents, and abilities I have that made those things happen for me. Then I would read that list to myself in the mirror. The first few times I read that I was generous, kind, or loving, I didn't believe it. Nevertheless, each day lovely moments would happen. After a couple of weeks of that, I could no longer deny it. I realized what I had never known before, that I am a unique, loving, generous, kind individual. I've gone through the Steps, so I see the change. I have not had the obsession to get high, and I have not burned my lips or had a black tongue in a few 24 hours.

I truly love Cocaine Anonymous. If it wasn't for the people who came in here and decided we could apply these principles to addiction, I'd be dead. That means something to me, and I'm really grateful. I now understand the concept of "the greater good" as reflected in Tradition One: "Our common welfare should come first; personal recovery depends upon C.A. unity." So how do I hold that unity? How do I make sure a meeting exists? How do I make sure that people consider the Traditions? How do I ensure that C.A. is going to be here for the newcomer? It's my responsibility, and for that I will show up.

From praying every day, from going through the Steps and applying these principles to my life, a change has occurred that has made me a really free and happy woman. And I know I'm not going to get high tonight. For absolutely sure, I am not going to get high tonight.

18

GOD SENT A TAXI

She took a ride home to Cocaine Anonymous.

I was an alcoholic by the age of six. Forced into the mother role after my parents divorced, I found that having a drink at the end of the day would take all of my problems away. Painkillers came shortly after the booze. It all worked well to get me out of reality.

By the time I was 12, I'd had enough of living with my mother. I got a full-time job and moved in with a couple, paying them for room and board. I went to school during the day, worked in the afternoon, and partied all night. It was then that I discovered my one true love—cocaine. I had finally found the reality-killer that I was looking for. It allowed me to use it and still be alert enough to continue in school and at work. I wasn't tired or hung over any more and, of course, no one could smell it on me. Cocaine got me to places I never imagined. I could go as high as I wanted without the fear of losing control. If I'd known where it was going to take me in the long run, though, I don't think I would have touched it.

My using went on until I was 20. I always had enough money and "friends" to keep me high. I went to the edge every day and always wanted to go further. The insanity was in my life long before I knew what it was. All my troubles were someone else's fault. "If they would only … " was a regular phrase out of my mouth. Just after my birthday, I embezzled money from the company I was working for. I was given probation and a strong warning to "straighten up." I was ordered to go to A.A.

In the small town I was living in, that meant going to the "old guy" meeting. I couldn't relate to any of them, and I didn't agree with their program of action, either. So I decided that if I had to sober up, it would be on my own terms. I went to about seven meetings in the next two and a half years. I stayed out of the booze and drugs, and I was definitely dry. My attitude and outlook on life didn't change a bit, though, and I still blamed everyone else for my woes.

Then came the day when I needed to use, or I thought I was going to lose my mind. My grandfather had died. Because I hadn't worked any of the Steps, I didn't know how to handle life on life's terms. I picked up and forgot my pain once again. That effect of the first hit would last four long years. The insanity returned. I couldn't do cocaine fast enough or long enough. My hits got bigger and bigger.

By this time I had a high-paying job that paid for everything I needed to stay high. It was the perfect job for an addict: I went on the road and could run away from myself every week. The only problem was that I kept finding myself everywhere I went. My boss was an addict as well (by his own admission), and since I was his best employee, I got special "snow bonuses." With a simple phone call I would get any drugs I wanted or the money to buy them. The party never stopped. I delegated all of my work to the people under me and kept using day after day.

I was given my own district office in the city where I wanted to move. I was tired of the road and looked forward to getting a life. At first things were okay. I would show up at the office, give orders, and then retreat to my personal office to commence with my daily ritual. I'd have my first hit to wake up, call the boss and tell him how good we were doing, and then use for the rest of the day. At night I would take the top guys out for a drink, and afterwards I would go home to finish what I had started hours earlier. My life seemed okay. Then it happened.

My employees got tired of the party life I had drawn them into. One by one they began to find their own things to do after work, and, in a few short weeks, I was left by myself at the end of the day. I fell into a deep depression that no amount of cocaine could kill.

Every day I fell deeper and deeper into a pit of hopelessness. I planned my suicide and then put the plan into action. I gathered the personal items I had taken to the office, said my regular good-nights, and left work for the last time.

My plan was to die before my next birthday, which was eleven days away. I wasn't going to leave a note or phone anyone. I was just going to take that one last hit, and it would be all over—just like that. All my pain would go away—just like that. I didn't, however, plan on the blackout I fell into.

I came back to consciousness three days after my birthday. I was so disappointed: I couldn't even kill myself properly. I continued to use, and it was soon the evening I was supposed to go to my grandparents' for the holidays. I called my family and told them the same "I'm sick" story that I had used for years. When I hung up, the reality that I was hopeless was overwhelming. I found every stash I had and put it all in one big hit. It was enough to kill an elephant. I hit it and waited for the silence. I slumped to the floor and waited. I couldn't move ... but I was still alive.

I got really mad at God then. I began to scream: "How could you? Why won't you let me die? What good am I?"

I took a few deep breaths and bargained for the last time. I told God that I was going to make two calls, one to my dealer and the other one to a detox. Whoever made it to my door first would win. If it were the dealer, God would let me go. If a cab showed up first, I would do whatever it took to sober up and change my life.

I made the call to my dealer, knowing that he only lived three blocks from me and would surely make it first. Then I called the detox. The woman who answered said it was a holiday and asked me if I wanted to wait until the next day. I told her that if I wasn't coming tonight, I wasn't likely to be alive tomorrow. She told me they had a bed and she would be waiting.

My next call was for a taxi. The operator thought I was crazy. She warned me that most people had made their taxi reservations weeks in advance for that night, but she said she would do her best to get me one as soon as possible.

Time crept forward. It seemed like minutes were taking hours as I watched the second hand move on my wall clock. Then the phone rang, and I almost jumped out of my skin. I picked the phone up with the anticipation of hearing my dealer's voice downstairs. I could have dropped dead right then: it was the taxi that I had called for. I put on my coat, went downstairs, and started on my journey to freedom.

I was introduced to Cocaine Anonymous through an H&I panel. Two guys came into the detox on a Saturday afternoon. They handed me pamphlets about finding *A Higher Power, The First 30 Days*, and one for newcomers. They shared what working the program in their lives had done for them and told us they got support from the Fellowship. They made it clear to me that going to meetings was a good start and that I should get a sponsor as soon as I could, a sponsor who had already gone through the Steps and could guide me through them.

Then they handed out meeting lists to everyone, and one of the members took my phone number. He said he would get in touch and take me to a meeting so I wouldn't have to be alone. There was something in his eyes that told me it was okay and that he wasn't trying to pick me up. When I got home a week later, there were several messages asking me to call him as soon as possible. I made the call and went to my first C.A. meeting that night.

I had finally found my home. As I sat and listened to the readings, I heard what I had experienced in the last months of my using. The paranoia, the carpet picking, and the sense that "they" were out there. Everything seemed to fall into place. I set out on what would soon prove to be the best choice of my life. I knew that night that I would never have to be alone again.

I found a sponsor within a few days. I went to four or five meetings a day, knowing they were the safest place for an addict to be. I commenced working the Steps. I had Step One down pat. I could see the unmanageability that was in my life and knew for sure that I was addicted to cocaine and all other mind-altering substances. I couldn't fool myself on that one. I couldn't even have one drink because if I did, my misery would come back tenfold.

Steps Two and Three were a bit tough. I had been to many churches in the past, and I never found a solution to any of my problems there. I had the idea that God was punishing and that He would bring me nothing but bad. My sponsor told me to ask my Higher Power to show me what He was.

That night I prayed for the insight I was looking for. I had a dream that took me back to when I was five years old. I had a childhood friend then who was invisible. He took care of me when I was scared, talked to me when I was lonely, and never let the bogeymen out of my closet. I realized the next morning that I had forgotten about him when I started drinking. I held on to him as my Higher Power. He was better than the concept I had of God from church, and he had never let me down when I was little. All I had to do was trust him again to care for me and guide me as I had let him before. It all became so simple.

Step Four was a long and painstaking process. I did what was suggested in the "Big Book," and my sponsor told me to do one column at a time so I wouldn't get overwhelmed. I read everything in the book on the Step and made sure I did all the inventories. Resentments were easy; my fears and sex conduct took a bit more effort, but in the end I did a thorough job on all of them. None of it seemed scary to me. I had realized that everything was in the past, and I just had to own it, accept it, and share it.

I was a bit apprehensive about Step Five. I scoured the rooms for someone I thought I could trust with my secrets. I listened intently to people when they shared. One night I went to a speaker meeting; the speaker had nine years sober, and he was sharing about what he said was the biggest gift of his recovery to that point. He had been an armed robber when he was out using. At the last bank he robbed, he had frightened a teller so badly that she'd wet her pants. At the time he saw this as his greatest accomplishment and had been very proud of it. In sobriety he met that woman again through a Public Information forum. He knew God had given him the opportunity to make amends. He talked to the woman afterward and asked for her forgiveness. She forgave him, and in that instant he felt God's presence. He realized that God had sent him a gift of His love that night, and it changed his life.

That was enough for me. If anyone would understand me, it had to be this guy. I wanted what he had, and I needed to share my story with him to find out how to get it myself. We made an appointment for the next day, and I shared everything with him. He shared more of his experience along the way, letting me know I wasn't the evil person I thought I was; I had been caught in the disease, and I could get well. I finally understood what I had been searching for all through my life: to be understood and to be loved unconditionally.

Willingness came easily for me in Steps Six and Seven. My earnestness for recovery had not dwindled one bit. I humbled myself to God and asked that He remove every one of my defects of character. Every word I said seemed to bring me more freedom.

I wrote down all of the names I had in my Fourth Step and added a few more. I prayed for the willingness to make amends to all of them. I knew that I could only benefit from making them. My life was getting better than I had ever imagined, and I wasn't about to put the brakes on and ruin what I had already received. I made direct amends to my family and wrote letters to the people who had died or that I couldn't find. I volunteered at community centers to make up for all the harm I had done to people I had never met. I also got a job and commenced making monetary amends. I was careful to not harm anyone by bringing up things they didn't know about; if they asked why I was doing things for them, I told them I needed to in order to heal my soul. I have not yet finished all of my amends, but I am doing my best to complete them as quickly as I created them.

I make sure I do a Step Ten inventory every night. I have found that over the years I have a shorter list all the time. God has removed some of my defects and made me very aware of the others. I take time every morning to thank Him for another day to do His will, and every night I pray for those still suffering that they may find Him, too. I also have a better understanding of others and myself today.

I try to pass on to everyone who has come to the Fellowship after me what was freely given to me by those who came before me. The

Promises have come true for me, and I have faith that they will come true for you. Give yourself a chance. Do the Steps, and find out how wonderful life can be: I promise you will find unconditional love, happiness, and freedom when you are done. God doesn't want us to be miserable or sick. Trust in Him, and trust in yourself. Ask for the help you need, pass it on to someone else, and you will be filled with a love you never knew existed.

19

A RECOVERED MISFIT

She discovered that her world was the right size and learned how to walk through rough times with dignity and grace.

All my life I felt empty inside. I felt like there was something missing in me, and everyone knew it. I felt like I never fit in anywhere. I spent most of my time going to great lengths to be the person I thought others wanted me to be. I was never any good at it, but I tried it over and over again.

As a teenager, I started drinking alcohol with my friends. I hated the taste, but I loved the effect it had on me. I couldn't see the point in ever having just one. One would not give me the effect I needed.

I got involved with the punk scene. I dyed my hair several different colors and wore all black. Finally, I felt that I had some kind of control. If I didn't fit in, it was because I chose not to. I was going to make the best of being a misfit. I used to think I was somewhat better than others were because I just drank and didn't do drugs. I remember being so excited because my friend had gotten some "fry" and it was "Fryday." And, oh, wasn't that just so cute? So on Friday we fried. On Saturday, I found out that "fry" was LSD. I thought, "Oh, my, if I did LSD, I might as well try everything else!"

That's the way my using always seemed to go. I would feel like I was somehow better than others (and somehow, not as good as them at the same time) because I didn't use what they used. Then they would say, "Want to try some?" and I would always take it. I hate to admit it, but I only did cocaine once. (Isn't that funny? Like I am ashamed I didn't do it more!) I stuck with all the "nonaddictive" drugs—you know, LSD; crystal meth; inhalants like rush, ether, and freon and drinking loads of alcohol. I used to be so proud of myself for never using crack or heroin. Looking back now, I realize it was never there. It was never in the same room as me, it was never offered to me. Had it been there, I really believe I would have tried it.

I found myself drinking more than I ever had before. I drank when I was depressed, when I was happy, when I was with friends, and when I was alone. Then crystal came back into my life. I only used on weekends at first. Well, maybe for the first two weekends. Then I was doing some after work. Then I did some more before work. Then I was doing it at work. I would stay up for days at a time and eat close to nothing.

I wanted to quit but couldn't seem to do it. I told this to one of my using buddies. He told me that he used to go to Cocaine Anonymous, how fun it was and how they really helped people who wanted to quit, and he offered to take me to meet a sober female friend of his. So we went, both of us high on crystal. To this day I don't know who that girl was, and I don't remember much about the conversation we had with her, but I do remember that she kept saying, "If you really want to quit, call your house right now and tell the rest of your using buddies to leave." I couldn't do it. They might not like me anymore! She told my buddy, "She's not done yet." I kept using after that, but the seed had been planted and started to grow.

My boss kept warning me that I was going to get drug tested, so I needed to cool it for a while or the big boss was going to fire me. I would promise her and myself that I was not going to use anymore. I meant it. With everything in me, I meant it. Then I would get home and one of my buddies would say, "Wanna line?" It would completely slip my mind that only 15 minutes before, I had made a vow never to do it again. I got drug tested. It was positive. My boss said if I ever tested positive again I would lose my job.

That same week the manager of my apartment complex came by and informed me that my neighbors were under the impression that I was running a crack house, and if I got one more complaint, I would be evicted. I thought this might be a good time to try one of those C.A. meetings my friend had told me about.

My using buddies told me about a real fun meeting that was just down the street and met every day at 4:45. I tried to get one of them to go with me, but they didn't want to get sober, so I went alone. I walked into the smoke-filled room, and a teenage girl walked up to me and asked if I was new. I burst into tears. She sat with me through the whole meeting. She encouraged me to get a newcomer chip. She gave me hope. That meeting gave me hope. I was afraid I was too young to get sober. I was only 24, but here was this 16-year-old staying sober and having fun.

I was afraid sober life would be boring, but these people were anything but dull. The jokes they made and the things they laughed at were sick—and I loved it. I know a lot of people in the Fellowship don't appreciate meetings where people are loud and obnoxious and yell things out during the readings. There have been times when I have felt the same way. However, I truly believe that had I walked into any other meeting, or any other Fellowship, I would not have come back. Not immediately, anyway. So, I try to remember that each meeting is autonomous and that it is that way for a reason. I believe my Higher Power led me to that kind of meeting because it was the kind of meeting I needed.

I kept coming back because it looked like they were having fun. People started hounding me to get a sponsor, so I did just to shut them up. I got nominated to chair the meeting for a month. Someone talked me into helping out on the Entertainment Committee. I started working the Steps.

When I was a kid, one of my chores was to vacuum the house. I hated to vacuum, but my parents would know when I didn't do it because there would be no wheel marks left on the carpet. So with my addict mind I would run the vacuum over the entire floor without turning the vacuum on. That is about the same way I approached the Steps the first time. I put more energy into trying to make people believe I was working the program than it would have taken to really work the Steps.

I stayed sober by the grace of God. I went to lots of meetings and did lots of service work. Finally, at about three years sober I was miserable. I started to really want what some of you had. I wanted to work the Steps again. I really wanted to work them this time. I have heard it said that when the student is ready, the teacher will appear. That was so true for me. I went to a meeting and heard a woman share about a Step workshop she was going to do. I jumped in with both feet.

I went through the "Big Book," turning the statements into questions and asking myself if I could relate. I would like to touch on a few key things that I learned in that process.

In Step One, I learned what an addict and/or alcoholic really is. I learned about the physical allergy. I looked back over my life and realized that normal people don't drink so much that they pass out in parking lots or in people's bathrooms on a regular basis. When I drank/used, it was for the effect it gave me. Whenever I picked up, I could never successfully predict when I would stop. I could intend to only have one drink or one line, but that rarely ever happened. I usually drank and used until it was gone. I learned about the mental obsession—how I would promise myself and anyone who would listen that I wasn't going to use again, and then someone would offer me a line and I would be off and running. You see, for the longest time I had doubts that I was really an addict/alcoholic. I kept hearing the war stories in meetings and could not relate. I did not go to prison; I didn't lose my home, my job, or my kids. But when I looked back over my life and saw my own experiences with the physical allergy and the mental obsession, I could finally admit to my innermost self that I am an addict and an alcoholic.

I always had believed in a Higher Power, I just never believed any Higher Power would waste His time on me. When I was on Steps Two and Three, I started noticing God in the rooms of C.A. I started noticing the way He was working in people's lives and slowly began to realize He was working in my life as well. I could be having a problem and I would go to a meeting and someone would be sharing how they had that same problem and how they got through it.

I had this ex-mother-in-law who hated me. She was such a witch. In doing Steps Four and Five, I discovered that she had every reason to hate me. First of all, when I left her son, I took everything my family had given us at the reception and left him everything his family gave us, which was nothing. Second, she "sold" me a car for $1,000, but she left the amount owed on the title blank. So I wrote "none" and never paid her. Those were a couple of pretty good reasons for her to dislike me.

I have learned from my experience that when I "work on" my character defects, they just get worse. God removes them for me, and He decides which ones need to go and when. My defects don't suddenly melt away because I am on Steps Six and Seven. They get removed in God's time. I usually don't notice right away when it happens, then one day I realize, "Hey, I am not obsessing about such and such anymore."

In preparing to make amends to my ex-mother-in-law, my sponsor suggested I should do two things. First of all, I needed to have at least half of the money I owed up front and make sure I paid the rest off in a timely manner. Next, I should listen for the Eighth Step sound. If I didn't hear it, I needed to hightail it out of there because I wasn't willing! I asked what the Eighth Step sound was, and he knocked on his desk and said "It's you knocking on her door with the money in your hand."

In preparation for my Ninth Step, I took out a loan for the full amount I owed her. I knocked on her door with the cash in hand. When she answered, I gave her the money and said, "I am an alcoholic and addict staying sober today on a spiritual basis. I can never get over drinking and using until I have done my utmost to right the wrongs I have caused people. I believe I have harmed you by hurting your son and never paying you for the car I got from you. I believe I owe you $1,000. It's all there." At that point she started crying and had to leave the room. When she returned I was sure she was going to try to get more money out of me or something. To my surprise, she never mentioned the money. She said, "My family is all that I have. When you hurt them, you hurt me." But it wasn't her voice I heard, it was my own mother's voice. My mother had said the same thing just a week or two before about someone hurting me. It suddenly hit me—this woman was no witch, she's just somebody's mom! I had no idea that I would be getting something out of making amends. Boy, was I wrong.

I have learned that working the Tenth Step on a regular basis keeps the size of my Fourth Step way down. It also helps keep me "right-sized." When I continue to see my errors, it's harder for me to think I am "better than" anyone.

I pray every day, but I have a hard time with the meditation part of Step Eleven. The more I try to quiet my mind, the louder it gets. So, I hear God's message through people at meetings, on TV, at work—I just have to listen.

I can't keep it unless I give it away. I have learned so many things as a result of working the Steps, and I learn so much by taking other people through the Steps. There really are no words to express the way my life has changed for the better. Oh, sure, there are the material things I have gained. I actually have a checking account, credit cards, a new car, a house, etc. I do enjoy them, but really, they are just things. What has changed the most, though, is me. I no longer feel like there is a huge hole in my gut. I feel as if it has been filled to overflowing with love and light and gratitude, and I know a greater happiness than I ever thought possible.

I am no longer alone, nor do I ever have to be again. I am so blessed to be a part of this Fellowship, to be among such incredible people. My Higher Power, the Steps, and the people in this Fellowship have been teaching me how to live, how to face life and all of its struggles, how to walk through the rough times with dignity and grace. I continue to learn and grow each day. I can never begin to repay what this Fellowship and my Higher Power have given me, but I hope to spend a lifetime trying.

20

LIVING LIFE TO THE MAX

Speeding through addiction, he surrendered to a new way of living, one day at a time.

I was born in Liverpool, the second son in a family of six children. My father was a dockworker who used to come home from work via the pub every night. My parents would fight physically, and more often than not, my dad would be so drunk that my mum would win. My elder brother used to climb out of the window and go to the phone box at the top of our street. Using a false name, he would call the police to report a disturbance at our address and then calmly climb back through the window and go to sleep. I swore I would never drink and I would never be like my dad. I was going to be a rock star or an actor instead. I didn't really care which—I just wanted to be rich and famous.

My best friend's dad was different. He owned the local chemist shop. My friend and I used to sneak his father's keys late at night, when everyone else was asleep. We would read from a big blue book, which listed illnesses of every kind and what drugs should be prescribed for each malady. It also listed the side effects of each drug. These side effects were of the most interest to us, and we experimented as often as we could. By the age of 15, I was also drinking alcohol because it brought on the side effects more quickly.

I left the family home at the age of 17 to work on the fairground. Phrases like "The louder you scream, the faster you go!" and "When the red light flickers, hold on to your knickers!" became my catch phrases, and my drinking became a daily habit. My favourite drug at that time was speed, which I had discovered in slimming tablets in earlier years. I loved it. On speed, I could drink as much as I wanted and never get drunk. I'd stay up for 70-odd hours at a time and then finally knock myself out with sleeping tablets on the third night.

Life was very full, and I could see no harm in living life with the sole purpose of enjoying every single minute of it. Of course, among the side effects of this lifestyle were waking up in police cells occasionally, or waking up with broken bones or other not-so-easy-to-fix ailments that required hospital treatment. Experiences such as these were "par for the course" or "occupational hazards," and I always bounced back very quickly.

I did everything very quickly. I lived in squats or stayed in the "Crazy Cottage" or the "Pirate Caves" at the fairground. Paying someone rent was not my style since I had much more important things to do with my money. I remember when someone brought a gram of cocaine over, I was totally unimpressed. "How much? £60 for that? You must be joking!" I didn't ask about, see, or hear about cocaine again until 10 years later.

I was eventually sacked from the fairground for gross misconduct. I claimed unfair dismissal and settled out of court. I was 20 years old and had fantastic, carefully thought-out plans for that money: A deposit for a house, a holiday, a new motorbike ... The money was gone in three weeks with nothing to show for it. All that was left were great stories of how I had spent it. Grandiose? Yes, I was.

I worked cash in hand for a rival fairground company to show the people who sacked me what a mistake they had made. I lost my license for drunk driving, and then heroin came to town. My dealer friends started to use it. The first time I saw someone inject it, my stomach turned, and I had to look out of the window to save myself from vomiting. Then the cat crept in and curiosity got the better of my common sense. I decided I wouldn't inject heroin, I would just chase it. I would only inject speed. That way, I knew I was not a junkie. I was injecting two or three grams of speed a day, chasing the dragon with smack, drinking alcohol, and popping pills, but my great mind told me that because I was not injecting the smack, I could not be a junkie.

Then I met the girl of my dreams and fell in love. We moved to London together, and she went to art school. I didn't know anyone to get drugs from, so I was clean, but I drank every day. And there were arguments. Within six months, I had hooked up with the local dealers, and within two years I was back into the needles.

The girl left me, and I lost my job and my home, so I went abroad to Turkey for a vacation. I got work playing guitar in beach bars. I had no drugs, so I just drank all day, every day. At the end of the season, they threw me out. A girl I had met in Turkey met me at the airport when I got home. She had been made redundant from a job, but she had cash. She bought me a new motorbike, and I stayed with her. She didn't do drugs, and she didn't know how much I had done in the past. She wouldn't have approved if I had told her, so I didn't. When she got pregnant, I demanded she have an abortion, but she would not.

I eventually got a job building loudspeakers. This got me access to all areas at concerts, and cocaine came back into my life. I was introduced to what I called "backstage champagne cocaine," and it was fantastic. I had arrived.

Over the next eight years, I used more and more. By now, I had three kids and lived in our family home with the girl from Turkey, whom I had married. I loved them, but I was more into impressing total strangers than showing an interest in my family's wants and needs. I preferred to stay at work, going home less and less. Work was far enough away from home that my wife believed me when I said I was working late and it was not worth coming home. When I did go home, I would try to sleep off the days I had been using at work. I had to drink heavily to knock myself out.

Although I never physically hit my wife or the kids, I was very controlling. They had to do everything I said to the letter, or I would fly off the handle and storm off to the pub. My wife had no idea I was using coke.

Eventually, my using was no longer backstage. I used alone, staying up all night at work looking at porn. I heard helicopters most of the night and looked through the gaps in the curtains for hours, thinking I was being watched. I was scared and paranoid, so I used more.

Money started to become a problem. All my credit cards were up to their limits, and I had taken out two large unsecured loans. I was also in the middle of applying for a second mortgage, but my wife knew nothing of my debts. I attempted suicide twice. I was laid off from work for a month to sort myself out. My boss told me that if I didn't slow down on my drinking, I was in danger of becoming an alcoholic. On top of it all, my elder brother, the one who used to climb out the window to call the police, died from a cocaine-induced heart attack. How could that be? He didn't use a fraction of the amount I used. We buried him, and I swore I would stop. I knew I was going to die if I didn't.

I went to meetings in another Fellowship and stopped using for a few weeks. I thought the people at the meetings were strange. They talked about God. "Get a sponsor, and work the Steps," they said. I didn't listen to them. I thought my problems were so much deeper than theirs and that they didn't understand. I started using again, and my wife found out about the money. Also, at a friend's house, she overheard me chatting up another woman while she and my kids were upstairs in bed. She filed for divorce.

I knew I had to stop, and I wanted to stop, but I tried and could not. My boss finally told me he had to let me go from my job, tears rolling down his face as he explained. I had used that morning, and although I didn't know it, that was to be the last time I used any mind-altering substance. I thought my life was over. I was not welcome at home or work and did not know where to go or what to do. The only place I could think of was a meeting, but I had tried that once, and it had not worked. Still, where else was there?

This time a lady at the meeting told me about Cocaine Anonymous. She told me of a local C.A. meeting on Sunday morning at 11:30. I went there, and I knew I had found home. The people there talked about using like I used. They said no matter how much they had, it was never enough. I saw people laughing about the chaos that used to be in their lives. I wanted to know how they were able to do that, and I felt the beginnings of hope.

I found out where more C.A. meetings were, and I went to them. I listened intently to what people said, but I had a great fear of asking anyone anything; my pride would not let me ask. But the feelings inside me grew, and the pain and torment of my past made suicide a daily consideration. I had to find someone to help me.

I asked somebody to be my sponsor, and he turned me down. I started to rant about him to the secretary of the meeting, when I noticed the secretary had the same spark in his eye that drew me to the other guy I had asked to sponsor me. I grabbed him and said, "Will you be my sponsor?" "Yes," he replied, "I would love to be your sponsor." Wow, what a relief! I told him I was on Step Four; I believed it because I had read the Steps on the wall and a bit in the literature. My new sponsor said, "Let's go back to Step One."

I had always felt different from others and now I knew why. I was a person who suffered from the disease of addiction. I had said so many times, "Yes, I'm an addict," or, "Yes, I'm an alcoholic," but I never knew what that those words really meant. Now I did. I learned I had to face the truth and admit to myself that I could not use because the allergy I have to mind-altering chemicals does not let me stop once I get started. I also learned I had a mental obsession that never lets me stay stopped whenever I try to stop. If I can't use because of my body and I can't not use because of my mind, then I know I am truly powerless over cocaine and all other mind-altering substances.

I was told gratitude is an action and not just a word, so I did service work from greeter to Group Service Representative (GSR). As GSR, it was suggested I learn about the Traditions. The Traditions are what keeps the group well. I have learned to use the Traditions not just in a group conscience and committee meetings but also in my everyday affairs. I have also done many other forms of service at the Area and Convention levels. I am a service junkie, and the feelings I get from helping others and doing service are the biggest buzz I have ever had.

I've learned to put the program first and work the program to the best of my ability on a daily basis. I put the program before my friends, before my job, before the car, before my wife and kids. I know that if I didn't, I wouldn't have any of the above. I would die, or even worse, go on living in the isolation and despair that had become my life.

I still have the same sponsor. I also have sponsees who bring me great joy as I work through the Steps with them. This causes me to look at the Steps on a regular basis to keep myself in check.

I have my old job back. At one year clean, I was convinced I had to leave my wife and kids, but I did not; it would have been running away, and I had done far too much of that in the past. I stayed, and my wife and I are working on our relationship. Without exception, the hardest place to work these Steps is in the home, but if I can't work them there, then working them everywhere else feels hypocritical. I have a wonderful relationship with my kids today. I feel the way I have wanted to feel my whole life—the feelings I had thought would come from using, or sex, or having money and prestige but never did.

Working the program in C.A. is enough for me. Through it I have access to a Power that enables me to live life, with all it has in store for me, without wanting to alter my mind. The Fellowship of Cocaine Anonymous, the Twelve-Step program of recovery and seeking God is what makes me feel whole and worthwhile as a person today. Deep down within me I know everything is going to be okay, and I know I need never use again so long as I carry on doing what I have learned. Today I live life to the max, one day at a time.

21

OUT OF THE STREETS AND INTO SOBRIETY

Recovery taught this former gangster how to give up, own up, make up and grow up.

As far back as I can remember, there was always a strange twist to my thinking. Most of the kids in my neighborhood had dreams of being baseball players, doctors, firemen, or President of the United States, things like that. Not me. I knew all my life what I wanted to be. I saw all the Cagney and Bogart films and knew them almost line for line. My role models were all around me. I'd sit on the steps of my building and watch the gangsters with awe. The street guys were my heroes, and I wanted what they had.

I found out early in life that if you want something, take it! Hit hard, hit fast, show no mercy, and the fruits of life would be mine. I had no time for school because it interfered with my dream. I quit school after the sixth grade and was hustling on the streets. That landed me six months in reform school, which is really a higher institution of learning the street life. When I was 14, I got sentenced to 18 months in reform school, and man, I was on my way!

Stick-ups, kidnapping, gambling, extortion, drugs, and con games were all good ways to make money, and I was raking it in. Years later, when I was getting sober, I realized that the lifestyle was harder to give up than the rock. The addiction to the lifestyle far exceeded the addiction to cocaine. As an adult, I did six and a half years in a maximum-security prison. By the time I crawled into the rooms of recovery, I had wasted eight and a half years behind bars. The sickest part was, I never thought there was anything wrong with that. I considered prison to be an occupational hazard, no more, no less.

I never considered myself an addict because I had it going on out there. I was truly living the dream I had always visualized. I was making big bucks, had lots of women, a wife and kids, and all the nice toys that money can buy. Who could ask for more? The answer to that, in case you're wondering, is an addict. Enough was never enough for me. I always had to have more: more money, more dope, more women, more power, more, more, more.

By the mid-1980s, my disease was in full swing. I had always liked the effect of anything that could take me out of reality. Cocaine was my lady, my lover. It was the truest relationship I'd ever had in my life. And boy, was I faithful! My cocaine habit was paramount. I gave up all other drugs except cocaine and alcohol.

Meanwhile, all around me my life was falling apart, and my small empire was crumbling. The money that came in wasn't being reinvested because I didn't have time. I was too busy with cocaine. I had a beautiful, faithful wife at home, yet night after night I was shacked up with other women, getting high. I found myself in the nastiest places in the city, whereas only months before I had owned a plush nightclub.

I was busy doing nothing, going nowhere fast, like a hamster on a wheel. There were 12 of us who dominated the streets, and we were widely feared and respected. Little by little, the others were getting busted or killed. Once, coming out of a four-day cocaine binge, I realized there were only three of us left. I had to sit down and make myself remember where the others were. Five were in prison serving 20 or more years and four were dead. I roused myself from the cocaine haze and tried to pull things together. After crashing for a good 10 hours, I told myself I needed to cut back on the cocaine and swore I wouldn't do any that day. For years, I had believed I could quit any time I wanted to, and that the reason I was still using was because I wanted to. It wasn't until I wanted to quit that I found out I couldn't. I left my house around midnight and went to an after-hours club. All I remember was ordering another drink. The next thing I knew, I was taking a telephone pole in half with my brand new luxury car about a block from my house. I had no memory of paying my tab, leaving the club, or driving to where

I hit the pole. That was a frightening experience, and I swore I would never drink again—without my cocaine.

Soon thereafter, I was arrested for a number of charges. It looked like I wouldn't see sunshine for many years, if ever again. I ran to my convenience-store God. (I only went there when I needed something.) I bargained and bartered with God that if He got me out of this one, I would change my life around. Though my money was getting short, I still had enough to live happily ever after. The trial lasted three and a half months, and miraculously, I was acquitted of all charges. It would be nice if I could tell you that's when I came into recovery, but I didn't even try to sober up. I forgot all about the deal I made with God. I thought I *was* God.

I went home, kissed the wife, hugged the kids, petted the dog, and got my pipe out. That started a two-year binge during which my wife left me after 17 years together. The law was all over me, and people were starting to think I wasn't so powerful any more. I said screw everybody and moved fifteen hundred miles away to a nice warm, sunny climate. All I wanted to do was hit the pipe and be left alone. After a year in my new town, I had gone through a small fortune in cash and property. The only thing I did each day was hit the pipe. I had smoked up a 17-year relationship and three huge money-making businesses, and I had kicked my kids to the curb, all for another hit. I believe that the end result of using is you wind up alone and hurting.

After a hard-working, innocent family man got busted for a kilo of cocaine that belonged to me, I found myself at a serious turning point. I knew I couldn't do cocaine any more, but I also knew I couldn't quit. My moment of clarity was that my life was crap. I was lost. I was so lost.

I can tell you a thousand insane stories about where this disease took me, but the bottom line is that the insanity of this disease is that I can't stop using. I don't want to do it, swear I won't do it, yet there I go, doing it again just like I swore I wouldn't. It was truly a hopeless state.

It was a few days before Thanksgiving when I crawled into the hospital, a broken man. If there was a light at the end of the tunnel, the bulb must've been out, because I couldn't imagine ever getting out of the hole I had dug for myself. All those old gangster movies ran through my mind, and I realized something that I never noticed before, even having seen some of them dozens of times. In the end, they *always* got killed or went to prison. Somehow, that seemed to fit where I was at right then.

My first spiritual experience came after about 10 days in treatment. I realized I hadn't had a drink or drug for those 10 days and that it was the first time in 21 years I had gone more than 24 hours without a chemical. If that's not a spiritual experience, I don't know what is.

I hear people share in the rooms a lot about relapse being part of recovery. I understand that's their experience, but it isn't mine. I was a straight-up dope fiend who would rip your heart out for another hit, but I have been sober ever since that first day. Relapse doesn't have to be part of recovery. If this is your first time trying to get sober, ask someone who understands the program of recovery to sponsor you. I was told to do what that person told me to do, if for no other reason than because it's not my own idea. If I'm beat up enough, I'll buy the concept that my way doesn't work. If I truly buy that concept, then I must believe I need some help. If I think I don't need to be told what to do, then I'm not completely giving myself to this simple program. I tried everything humanly possible not to wind up here, but here I am. There must be a God in charge.

This is how it happened for me. The first three Steps taught me how to give up. Four, Five, and Six taught me how to own up. Seven, Eight, and Nine taught me how to make up. Ten, Eleven, and Twelve taught me how to grow up. I worked Steps One, Two, and Three and got right with God. I worked Steps Four, Five, and Six and got right with myself. I worked Steps Seven, Eight, and Nine and got right with you. Steps Ten, Eleven, and Twelve help keep me right with God, with me, and with you.

I sit here today with over 13 years of sobriety. I've learned how to apply these principles in life and have been successful in business. Today I'm a productive member of society. In recovery I have earned a master's degree and regained my voting rights. I have a passport today (a real one) and have traveled all over the world. What a blast hitting meetings and conventions in other countries! I look back at being a kid sitting on the steps daydreaming, and it seems like a different lifetime. How fortunate we are to be given a whole new life, a whole new chance to live. Going from the end of a gun barrel or a crack pipe to a recovering member of Cocaine Anonymous seems like a fairy tale come true. All I have to do is suit up and show up, be available to those who need help, keep working the Steps, and anything is possible.

22

LIFE LESSONS

Facing challenges helped her find the strength and faith to follow her calling.

I grew up in a large family on a farm. My father died when I was eight, so I was raised by my mother. My first experience with alcohol was not significant. I never drank socially. I always drank to get drunk, just like everyone else I hung around with. I had a turbulent adolescence, moved out of my mother's home, and dropped out of high school at the age of 16. I moved in with a couple who owned a bar, and I began to drink daily. I was experiencing blackouts when I was 16, so when I found cocaine, I thought it was wonderful. Not only did it help me stay thin, I could drink without going into a blackout every time.

My drinking and using progressed over the years. I used cocaine for 10 years until I went to treatment. When I was 25, things started to fall apart. I was writing bad checks to pay for everything and using my cash to pay for my drugs. The bad checks started a cycle of arrests. Being arrested didn't really faze me; I have been arrested more times than I care to count. I wound up getting two tickets for drunk driving (DUI) within three months and finally started to hit bottom.

A big part of my bottom was the isolation from my family. We have experienced enough tragedy to be very close. My sister has always been my best friend. We had also partied together, but as my using progressed, there was something different about my behavior. I ended up avoiding my family as much as possible.

When I didn't show up for court on my DUI, a warrant was issued for failure to appear, and I was arrested at work. I remember it very clearly because it was my mother's birthday, and, once again, I hadn't shown up when I said I would. I lost my job, and that was the beginning of the end. Now I was homeless, unemployed, and had serious legal problems. And I was totally delusional: I still didn't really connect my problems with the drugs.

I was scheduled to be in court in two different towns at two different times. I called my sister, and we rode around drinking while I told her about my predicament. My solution was to leave town. She suggested that I go to this local treatment center, get off the cocaine, and give my mother some time to straighten out my legal problems. The treatment center had a swimming pool, and I guess that I thought I was going on vacation. I packed a grocery bag with a few clothes, some skimpy shorts and my bikini, and went to treatment.

I didn't know anything about treatment. I had no idea that they were going to ask me to quit drinking. I cried most of the first two weeks. They kept saying that I was a little girl who needed to grow up and that my family was going to kill me if they kept enabling me. They taught me about the disease of addiction and said that if I wanted to get off the coke, I had to quit drinking as well.

They talked about the Twelve Steps and gave me assignments to start on them. When I saw the word "God," I realized I was angry at God. I had been taught that you have to do some specific things in order to get to heaven, and my father hadn't done any of those things. I didn't want to have anything to do with a God that would take away a little girl's father and not let him go to heaven. I also knew that I could not live up to the standards of my religion.

So I decided to test God. The treatment counselors had suggested that I go to a halfway house to get a solid foundation of recovery after treatment. I will always remember going to my room and telling God, "If you are there, I need you to let me know. And I need it to be clear that I need to go to a halfway house, not just these counselors telling me."

The next day I received a book of stories. I scanned the contents and started reading one of them. I started crying. The woman in the story was the same age as I was at the time, came from the same size family, and was born the same day I was. In the story, her treatment center wanted her to go to a halfway house. It was the same halfway house I was being told to go to. I knew then that God was letting me know that He was there for me.

I called my mother and told her that they wanted me to go to a halfway house, and she said, "Thank God." Going to a halfway house was the best thing I could have done for my recovery. For three and a half months, all I had to do was focus on my recovery. I didn't know anyone, so it forced me to reach out to people in the Fellowship. I started tagging along with people with long-term sobriety, and I found out that I didn't need an invitation to go with everyone for coffee after meetings. It was a great experience. I worked the Steps and had a wealth of experience to pull from. These people taught me about the Traditions and how we can only be torn apart from within. They reinforced the need to give back to the Fellowship and explained to me my responsibility to ensure that the Fellowship is here for the next addict.

My first year was almost magical. I learned to ask for help. I accepted that I am an alcoholic as well as an addict. I faced all of my legal issues and started to make amends, and I decided not to return home. I found the willingness to go to any lengths, primarily because I knew that God was there for me. Prayer became one of my most valuable tools.

Cocaine Anonymous started in my area the year before I got sober, but I didn't really get involved for a couple of years. At first, I couldn't bear to hear people talk about cocaine. I got involved in C.A. during my third year of sobriety and have been active ever since. I've had the honor of holding every position of service from ashtray washer and greeter to Area Delegate. Every position has been a great experience.

I went back to school and got my bachelor's and master's degrees, although life continues to teach me that who I am has nothing to do with the initials behind my name. Recovery has allowed me to surpass all my dreams. My husband and I decided to travel and chose London as our first destination. We attended the Cocaine Anonymous U.K. convention several years ago and were so warmly welcomed; we were taken into people's homes and made immediate friends. I have no doubt that I made lifelong friends during that trip. My whole understanding of the Fellowship changed then, which is part of the reason that I am so committed to my Area and our Region. It helped me really grasp that we are part of a much larger picture.

Sometimes God doesn't let me see the whole picture because I would never go along with certain ideas if I knew all the details at the beginning. For example, that trip made me stop and look at my life. Somewhere along the way I had gotten caught up in the belief that more is better, still judging success by financial standards. In fact, all that belief was doing was adding stress to my life. There were so many lessons for me in facing that. And my challenges over the years have taught me other hard lessons. A very wise woman once told me, "Our challenges don't mold our character, our challenges reveal our character."

Certain life lessons keep rotating through my life, and I recognize them more quickly each time. I have learned that there is a beginning and end to everything, and I can embrace change. My challenges help me become a more compassionate person and to be of greater service. I've learned to keep my eye on God's plan, not mine, that my choices and behaviors need to reflect my priorities and values, and that out of everything I perceive to be negative, something incredible emerges.

Life continues to teach me what it really means to be a responsible member of society and to be of service to the suffering addict. I have finally found the strength and the faith to follow my calling regardless of where it takes me, who is with me, and who disagrees. I finally understand that it is not my job to fit in. The challenges that I face are present to teach me something that is necessary for my continued usefulness. I love this Fellowship and the way of living that it has given me. I trust that the best years of my existence lie ahead.

23

AN ULTIMATUM TO GOD

"Just say no" and "Just don't pick up" did not work for this addict. She finally heard the message while listening for God to answer her challenge.

As you read my story, I hope you will focus on the similarities between us and not the differences. Looking at the differences nearly killed me. I spent most of my life constantly comparing my insides to your outsides, the way I felt to the way you looked.

I was born the middle child to an average, lower-working-class Canadian family. The big family outing was going to church every Sunday, where my grandparents, aunts, uncles, and cousins all met us. Though I was part of a large family, I did not feel I belonged.

We did not have a TV or carpet on the floors or fancy clothes. I was dressed in homemade or hand-me-down clothing. My father worked two jobs to support the family but still found time to play and teach us biking, swimming, baseball, and fishing. I was loved and cared for and did not lack the attention of very caring parents.

I did not like school at all. I was teased by classmates about my clothes, shoes, and hairstyle. It made me feel very uncomfortable and dissatisfied with our station in life. I kept much to myself. I liked to play alone and use my imagination. I felt that I was different and did not fit in the school world.

My world as I knew it was blown apart when my parents divorced, something which surprised me because I never noticed any discord between them. Perhaps I was already too self-involved to notice their troubles. Divorce was a dirty word. It was hushed up and nobody talked about it. My feelings of being different and not good enough were reaffirmed.

My mother, brother, sister, and I moved in with my grandparents. I was very unhappy and missed my dad. I changed schools and again viewed myself as a social outcast. I began to hang out with a group of misfits who were inhaling nail polish remover and glue to get high. I tried it. I liked it. Soon, I was doing it daily. I was nine years old, and I was arrested for the first time in my life while using in the park.

My mother remarried, and we moved again. Another new house, new school and new neighbourhood. Now I also needed to compete for attention with four new brothers and sisters and a new stepdad. Although the neighbourhood was better, the combined family crowded the home. My sister, brother, and I lived in the basement, while my stepbrothers and stepsisters had their own rooms.

Now I really felt different, not good enough, and not a part of. I began to drink and smoke pot. Upon entering junior high, I became sexually active. Drugs, sex, and alcohol allowed me to numb the feelings of being not good enough. I became disruptive in school, and the school board recommended that I get special help.

I was sent to live in a convent for the next 18 months. My parents had high expectations. They had spent good money to change my bad-ass attitude and instead got a more refined bad ass. My stepfather was an impatient man, beating me when he lost his temper. I was angry with my mother for not protecting me. At the age of 15, I decided to move out.

I lied about my age to get a job. I worked by day and partied by night. Free love was the buzzword of the era, and I thrived on the attention. My life was out of control. When I finally burnt out, I moved back home.

On my return home, I found out I was pregnant. I decided to have an abortion under pressure from my parents. I felt a very real and deep sense of loss, guilt, and emotional pain. I tried to go back to school, but I thought I was "grown up" and couldn't relate to the other kids. I took a trade course and excelled, focusing on an area that gave me a great deal of satisfaction.

I began dating an older, mature man, and we moved in together. We partied and drugged for the next three years. Then we got married, and everything changed. I stopped doing drugs, bought a house, had a baby, and settled down. Life was very "normal."

But something was still missing. When I decided we needed a change, I asked my husband, "Do you love me?" He said "No." I had expected a different answer. My self-esteem was shattered. I felt betrayed. I was not going to stay in a loveless marriage, so I filed for divorce.

What does a single, 22-year-old woman with a one-year-old baby do? With money in the bank and a huge resentment toward my ex, I tried the bar scene. I began getting invitations to those parties after the bar closes where cocaine was abundant. I really liked the sensation that comes when chemicals numb reality. I liked the effect of cocaine so much that I began to do it at work, in the car, at family gatherings, and just about anywhere. I believed cocaine made my life better. I believed I was smarter, prettier, funnier, and more efficient.

I began to notice that there was something different about the way I did cocaine. Other people went home at the end of the evening. Other people were okay when there was no more left. I was not. My body had an insatiable need. I took drugs into my body, and I could not stop. I was embarrassed that I wanted more, so I sought out the people who partied like I did.

Within a year I began to use intravenously. My parties were different now—just the bag and me in a locked bathroom for hours or days until the cocaine ran out. I spent all the money I had saved, all the money I earned, and all the money I was getting from my boyfriends and ex-husband. I used as much and as often as I could. Cocaine was my master, and I would do anything to get it. I sold everything I had, including my body. If the dealer would have taken body parts, I would be short a few fingers and toes today.

As my disease progressed, my behaviour became more excessive. I lied, cheated, conned, and manipulated people. I hated who I had become. I dragged my daughter through it all. Somehow, I managed to keep my job. It probably kept me in denial longer because I thought that if I can get up and go to work, I must be all right.

I lived the Jekyll and Hyde life for years. My daughter and I moved from place to place and from man to man, choosing partners for what I could get from them.

Finally, I moved back home with my parents and there tried commit suicide. They called a doctor to examine me. He pulled up my shirtsleeves, and my mother saw the deep bruises and track marks on my arms. She was shocked. I was ashamed. I wanted to quit for my family but did not know how. I went to a treatment program but did not complete it. I was using again the following week.

I decided that I had to find new ways to hide my using. I worked during the day and used at night. I tried only using on weekends and believed that it hardly ever interfered with my work. Sometimes I could go a whole week without using, but the weekend always found me in my favourite places, the bathroom or the dealer's house. Although I knew cocaine was hurting my family and was physically, emotionally, and financially draining me, I had to have it. I knew by this time that I was hopelessly addicted.

Over the next 10 years, I remarried twice. There were many affairs and many nameless men. I traded myself for rent, drugs, food, alcohol, and money. Many well-meaning family members, boyfriends, and husbands tried to help me quit. I visited detoxes and hospitals so many times I could not keep track. Once I was hospitalised for three months with gangrene and nearly died. The hospital placed a shunt in my arm to administer medication for the wound in my leg. I went home and swore I would never use cocaine again. Three days later, I found it was convenient to use the shunt for shooting dope. I had promised my daughter, my family, myself, and even God that I would not use again, and yet I could not stop.

I continued to use, and things continued to get worse. I had to have it. I watched using friends die. I lost friends, family, and material things. I had lost my pride, my self-esteem, and my faith.

By some miracle, I ended up in a Twelve-Step meeting with a friend of mine who had asked me to support her. I listened to people sharing and heard some similarities. Though I was not yet ready to acknowledge my addiction, the seed was planted. The people I saw were smiling and laughing, and, most important, sober. Of course, I thought most of them were lying, but they had a certain appeal. They seemed to be doing something right.

I went to meetings for four years and never achieved more than 10 months of sobriety. Each time I returned more ashamed. As strange as it may seem, though, I kept coming back.

The last time I used drugs, I had overdosed at the end of a five-day run. All was black when I slowly came to. My daughter was outside the bathroom door, crying softly, "Mommy, please come out. Mommy, please don't die. Mommy, I love you."

The last thing I remembered, I had been at the dealer's house, doing drugs in the bathroom. Feelings of pain, guilt, fear, remorse, terror, and sadness began to poke through my drug-induced numbness. I was broken spiritually, emotionally, mentally, physically, and financially. I saw no way out. How did a nice girl like me end up a junkie in the bathroom? I had been to enough Twelve-Step meetings that I was not enjoying drug use at all anymore, yet I could not rid myself of the obsession.

When all the drugs were gone, I let my daughter in. She bathed me and put me to bed where I lay sobbing. I was beaten. I remembered a friend had suggested that I pray and ask for help. I had not prayed before because I did not believe in God, so how could I pray to God for help? Now I was willing to do anything, and I had that little seed of hope that it might help. So I gave God an ultimatum: show me a way out within the next 24 hours, or I will kill myself.

The next day I went to a Twelve-Step meeting and listened to the message I had probably heard a hundred times before. For some reason, this time the words went from my head straight to my heart. In that instant, I began to understand the simplicity of this Twelve Step program. I finally understood that all I had to do was stay sober today, one day at time. I began taking suggestions, praying, and going to meetings, one day at a time. It made such a huge difference.

I was excited to try more suggestions that would change my life. The same friend who suggested I pray recommended that I go to a Cocaine Anonymous meeting. At the time, there were only three C.A. meetings in the local area, but I sought them out and went regularly. During that first meeting, I heard the reading *Who is a Cocaine Addict?* and knew I had found a home. This was to become my C.A. home group. I got a sponsor. I began to work the Twelve Steps. I could finally talk about my problems with people who understood. As I worked the Steps, I found a new sense of freedom unlike anything I had ever known.

Working the first three Steps, I began to understand the fatalness of my disease and that I could not stop on my own. I know now why phrases like "just say no" and "just don't pick up" do not work for addicts like me. I am completely without defence from the first hit. On my own, I lack the power to stop and stay stopped. So where was I going to find the power to stop and stay stopped? Step Two proposed that either God was everything or God was nothing. I was left to choose, and the answer would help me stop using drugs.

Step Three has been a process for me over the years. Being a selfish, self-centred addict, it is difficult for me to entirely turn my will over to God all at once. I came to understand that I only had to make the decision. The rest of the Steps would help me carry out that decision.

In Step Four I began to see how nearly all my actions had placed me in positions to be harmed. I no longer had to blame the rest of the world for all my misery, and I could fix the root of my problems since they centred in me and not others. This was very freeing. I found it impossible to be a victim after doing a thorough Step Four.

In Step Five, I released many of my long-held fears by sharing them with God and another human being. My many fears and phobias seemed to slip away. Suddenly my life was taking on new meaning and joy, and I was barely halfway through.

After reviewing the first five Steps, I thanked God from the bottom of my heart and prayed for the willingness to have my defects of character removed. In Step Seven, I humbly asked God to remove my shortcomings. I found that I could neither wish nor will these things away. I had to be willing and follow through with the remaining Steps.

Steps Eight and Nine are an ongoing process. My list of people I had harmed fell into three categories. The first group of amends I was willing to make immediately. The second group I was either unable or not quite ready to do. The third group was the "not on your life" category. I know that I will not be entirely free until I have done my utmost to right the harms I have done others. I know that many an addict finds his way back to the pipe, needle, or straw because of not following through with the Ninth Step. Most of my first two categories of amends are done. Some of the "not on your life" amends are done, and nearly all have moved up to the willing category. Making amends has allowed me to hold my head high and look people in the eye without fear. When I find myself balking at the Steps, especially the Ninth Step, I am reminded of my sponsor's words, "How free do you want to be?"

Steps Ten and Eleven are part of my daily life today. It is my habit now to review each day and see where I have harmed someone or been self-seeking or dishonest. If I am wrong, I have learned to admit it. This was not always an easy proposition for me, but through my years, I have found that if one is going to eat crow, it is best to do so when it is young and tender.

I seek to better understand my Higher Power through prayer and meditation. Today, I know that quiet contemplation works for me. I find quiet time at the beach or near the water to work best. I need not be in a church or a specific place to pray or meditate.

Working the Twelfth Step has brought such joy to my life that I find it difficult to describe all the gifts I've received. Practicing the principles of the Twelve Steps and carrying the message of C.A. have become passions in my life. When I was 30 days sober, I went to my first detox meeting as a member of C.A. and not a client. I saw how we can touch each other's lives and share our experiences, even if we have only a few days more sobriety than our fellow addict. Only those who have been literally saved from the pain of addiction can relate and win the confidence and trust of another addict. The concept of one addict working with another is one of the greatest gifts of the Twelve Steps of Cocaine Anonymous. I have found that I cannot keep this priceless gift of sobriety unless I give it away.

Being of service to this Fellowship of C.A. is one of the greatest gifts given to this addict. I have held many service positions from the Group and Area level to the World Service level. It is truly a spiritual experience. What I have received in return are more friends than I could possibly have imagined from all over the world and all walks of life and the peace of mind that comes from doing for others.

I came to C.A. for one thing, to stop using cocaine. I carried a lot of baggage and some unimpressive credentials. I stayed and worked the C.A. Steps and found a Power greater than myself, greater than cocaine. Today I am a mother, sister, employer, sponsor, and friend to many. I enjoy real life today. I dance, I pray, I laugh, I work, I love. I live life as it happens in the present, not yesterday or tomorrow, but fully in the moment. Is my life perfect? No. Have I become a perfect human? No. Just perfectly human, and that's progress for this cocaine addict.

24

IN SPITE OF MYSELF

It worked because she worked the Steps.

I thought I was raised in a pretty normal family. My dad was an alcoholic who left my mother when I was one year old and my sister was just born. For years it was just my mom, my sister, and me. During that time my mom never drank, did any drugs, or even smoked a cigarette. I thought life was great and that's how everybody's life was.

Life took a dramatic change when I was 10 years old and my mother met my stepfather. My mom started partying and would leave on Friday, and my sister and I wouldn't see her until Sunday. When I was 11 years old, my stepfather began molesting me, and I started to withdraw from everything. I was introduced to alcohol and pot when I was 13, and I realized that if I stayed wasted, I didn't have to feel the pain and could escape the misery that my life had become. I smoked pot, popped pills, and drank as much as I could get my hands on. It worked for the next 18 years.

When I was 15 years old, I told on my stepfather, and the police came and picked up my sister and me from school. In court, the judge told my mom to divorce her husband or give up custody of her children. She decided on the latter, so my dad took us. I didn't know at the time that my dad was a drunk. I was just so relieved to not be in that situation with my stepfather any more.

At that point, I still believed that everything bad that had happened to me and everything bad that I had done in my life was my stepfather's fault. I blamed all my behavior and drug problems on being sexually abused. The funny thing is that when I was removed from that situation, my disease followed me.

I graduated high school somehow, partying through all of it. I smoked cocaine for the first time, and I really liked it. Then I didn't do any more for a year. Never even thought about it. During that time I met my future ex-husband. We had a daughter, and I stayed home with her, and he worked. We bought our pot from a guy who taught us how to mix it with rock cocaine to make a primo. Oh, man, I was in love with those. We had ourselves a little primo problem for a while. Some nights we would go to the dealer's hotel and smoke with him for hours. While we were there, we would put our little girl in her carrier and put her over in the corner, thinking we were good parents by trying to keep her from getting a contact high. We started pawning things. Soon we had nothing. We decided we needed to stop. I mustered up some self-will and quit ... only the primos, though.

Our daughter was three when we split up, and all hell broke loose. My ex-husband took her from me and threatened my life on a regular basis. The only way I knew how to deal with all this was to get high, so that is what I did. I finally let him have custody of our daughter.

When I met my current husband we were both wasted. That is how our marriage would be for eight years. We spent all our time getting wasted, beating the crap out of each other, breaking everything in the house, and making up the next day.

During all this mess, my ex-husband was dealing crack, and we would smoke with him for hours. My husband was still able to go to work and pay the bills, but I was only able to smoke crack cocaine. One weekend I stayed with my ex and his new girlfriend smoking, and my little girl was there the whole time. On that Sunday my ex went crazy and left the state with my daughter. He left me there with no money, no food, and—worst of all—no dope. I went crawling home. My husband took me back, but said we had to stop the cocaine, and I couldn't see my ex or my daughter. I agreed. Once again, I mustered up enough self-will to quit the cocaine only.

I started working and tried to go on with my miserable life. One night my husband and I got very drunk, and once again we beat the crap out of each other. This time I was knocked unconscious. The next day I vowed that I would never drink again. Again, I used some self-will to stop drinking, but I still smoked pot and popped a valium here and there.

Then I got pregnant. I had been trying to for some time and was very happy. One night my husband came home drunk and got very mean. I told him he had to quit drinking, or I was leaving. He quit, and we got ourselves together a little. We bought a nice house, brand new cars and trucks, four-wheelers and dirt bikes, and we had a beautiful son. Although we were still smoking pot and popping the occasional pill, life was wonderful for the first time in many years.

I became involved with church. I went there high on pot and pills, and even though I was not living any spiritual principles in my life, I thought I was doing good because I went to church on Sundays. During all these years my relationship with my mother had been on again, off again. I hated her husband and hated her most of the time. Then one night I had what I now refer to as a spiritual experience, and I forgave my stepdad. Shortly after that, he became very ill with cancer. We started to spend a lot of time together. (Don't get it twisted, though; every time I went to spend some time with him, I would steal his valium and oxycontin.) When he got really bad, I started to pray. I begged God to spare the person I had spent years hating. He died anyway, and I developed a giant resentment toward God. I also picked up the pipe again.

Things went downhill quickly after that. My husband and I smoked, shot, and snorted as much cocaine as we could. We started to lose everything. We would get our dope, go into our room, shut the door, and get high. I had no idea what my children did for dinner or how they bathed themselves, and I really didn't care as long as they left me alone. Sometimes we would put them to bed and leave for the whole night. The house could have burned down, and we would have never known it until we got home. We smoked up all our possessions, everything in our house, and then we smoked up the house. It's amazing what you can fit on the end of a crack pipe.

I got pregnant again right before we lost our house. At first I was in denial; I thought I was just partying too much, and my body wasn't right, but I was pregnant. When I was about three months along, I went into cocaine-induced convulsions. I decided then that I wasn't going to smoke any more crack cocaine. I wanted to stop using through my entire pregnancy, but that little bit of self-will I was able to muster up before was completely gone. No matter how much I wanted to stop, I could not. No matter how much I knew I needed to stop, I could not. You haven't seen anything until you've seen a woman eight months pregnant crawling around on the floor for hours looking for dope that isn't there.

The last time I got high, I had been up for three or four days when my water broke. Normally this would be a joyous occasion, calling the family, getting bags ready, stuff like that; it was not so for me. I did not want to go have this baby. I knew in my heart it was going to be bad. I waited as long as I could before I went to the hospital. When my son was born, he was shaking violently. He went into a neonatal intensive care unit.

The day after I had him, the doctors, nurses, police, and government social workers came into my hospital room. They told me there was cocaine, marijuana, and xanax in my son, and that he wasn't going home with me. They said that I had a problem and needed to do something about it. I told them that I didn't know what had happened, that there must have been a mistake. They looked at me like I was crazy. They also took our other kids.

The only thing I knew about recovery was that my dad got sober in another Fellowship. My husband and I went to our first meeting. I was very scared and nervous. When I said that I was an addict, I was asked to leave. I thought, "Oh, my God! Even these people don't want me." But a lady there told me about Cocaine Anonymous. My husband and I went to C.A. that night and went back every night. We would drive for 45 minutes just to get to the meetings and 45 minutes to get back home.

I had no intentions of getting a sponsor or working any Steps. I was only going to do what I was told by the courts so I could get my kids back and go on with my life, even though it was falling apart. I had absolutely no faith in this program ... some literature, Twelve Steps, and a room full of dope fiends? Please. My social worker wanted the name and number of a sponsor, so I said, "Crap, I guess I'll get one." Then it was all about, "What if that social worker calls and that sponsor says I haven't done anything?" I had barely enough willingness to work the Steps. In spite of myself, I started changing and so did my life.

When I got here I thought cocaine was my problem, but in working the Steps with my sponsor, I learned so much more. I learned why I do cocaine even when I don't want to do cocaine. I learned why I can't stop once I start. I learned a lot about this disease, but most importantly, I learned about myself.

I emphasize working the Steps with a sponsor for a reason. I believe that if I had tried to work the Steps on my own, I would not have gotten anything out of this program and would probably be dead today.

My life has changed in so many ways. When I got here I couldn't stand God and thought He couldn't stand me. Today I have a God in my life that I love and that loves me, no matter what. Do not get it twisted; everything in this program has taken a lot of work for me. It has taken a lot of action, even when I didn't want to do it.

Improving my life with my family has taken the most work. One day I woke up next to a stranger—my husband. I had no idea who he was because we spent the first eight years of our marriage messed up. At first I wasn't real sure if I liked him very much sober. We have put a lot of work into our marriage, and it is getting better. Now we have been together a little over 11 years, and we are still working on our relationship today.

When I got sober, I had two teenagers who were used to being their own parents. All of a sudden, I wanted to be their mom and wanted to know what they were doing and who they were doing it with, all those questions "normal" parents ask. This has taken a lot of work also, and we are still working on it today.

My baby had a lot of medical problems because of my selfishness. His body was stiff, like when we are tweaking out and our jaws get tight and we tense our whole body; his body was like that all the time. They told me that he might not ever sit up or walk, and that if he did walk, it would be with braces on his legs. He has had a lot of physical therapy and a lot of speech therapy. He wears glasses and has tremors. When he is concentrating on something, his hands will shake. But I don't have to live in the "Oh, my Gods!" anymore. I know today that I can be there for my son.

I also realized that life still happens even though I stopped drinking and using. My grandmother was diagnosed with breast cancer when I first got into recovery. I didn't have to use behind it, and I could actually be there for my family. My dad got very sick and almost died this year, and I spent every night at the hospital with him. I didn't have to go use behind that, either.

I have experienced having a child in sobriety. Even though I had been pregnant several times before, I had never done it completely sober. What an experience that was! When my child was only three weeks old, he stopped breathing. I had to give him CPR and we rushed him to the hospital. At first all I could think of was, "Why me? I'm being good, doing what I'm supposed to do, why is this happening?" I called some people in the Fellowship, and they had to remind me that I was sober and able to be there to save my child's life. You see, if it had happened when I was still using, I would have come out of my room from getting high to find a dead baby on the couch. But I didn't have to use behind my child getting sick; I could be there for him.

I can be there for all my kids today. I know what my children had for dinner and that they had baths. I can pay my bills when they come in the mail, I haven't had to go to the pawnshop in quite some time, and the only time I crawl on the floor today is to pick up toys.

The Fellowship of Cocaine Anonymous is amazing. When I first got there and everybody was laughing and cutting up, I thought, "What the hell is so funny? If you knew where I just came from, you wouldn't be laughing." I didn't know that they did know where I had just come from, that they had been there, too. People from that group have sat with me for hours in a hospital room. The women have brought meetings to me when I couldn't get to meetings. They are amazing. I have relatives, and I have my family—my family is the people in Cocaine Anonymous.

Because of Cocaine Anonymous I have a life. I can live life on God's terms. I am happy, joyous, and free. I work with others and stay very involved in service work at a Group level, at a District level, and now at the Area level. Today when I tell people that I am going to do something, they know that I will.

I see a lot of people come in and out of the rooms. Today I am not willing to risk it. I know that I have to keep doing what I have been doing: meetings, the Twelve Steps, work with my sponsor, service work, all of it.

When I was out there using, I was willing to go to any length to get what I wanted; I would have given you my right arm for another hit of dope. Today I am willing to go to any length for my recovery. Even if you don't think this thing will work for you, if you give it a try, your life can't help but change. Mine did, in spite of myself.

25

MY FOREVER CLEVER MIND

The simple concept of one addict helping another proved far more effective than his own best thinking.

It's another Sunday morning, and I'm not trying to escape what I did Friday and Saturday night. I simply woke up this morning. Actually, the birds woke me up, and it was beautiful hearing birds. Which is a change because if you're an addict like me, you know all about getting ticked off at the birds first thing in the morning.

If you're an addict like me, you have a mind that sometimes forgets everything. I've got a forever clever mind that's like a steel colander. Stuff just goes right through it all the time. Drugs work the same way; they always wore off, and I was left with myself. I found that even in recovery, it's the same. So, I need to do this thing daily, and I'm grateful that it works that way.

I grew up in a family that gave me all the love and support I could ever want. I never went without, and I'm deeply grateful for that. Despite all I had, I never quite felt comfortable inside of myself. I had those feelings like I never quite fit in, like I could never really match up to you, and that if you really knew me, you wouldn't like me. I could not put a finger on any of these feelings until I got here and started doing the work. It wasn't like, "I don't feel adequate. Pass me that joint." It was never a conscious thing. On a conscious level, I got loaded because it felt good. That's all I knew, man.

Books were my first escape, but nothing worked quite like that first beer. I don't know exactly why I drank it. Today I have some hunches. Uncomfortable and teased as a kid, I saw adults sitting around drinking and smoking pot. When I got my opportunity, I stole a beer out of the fridge. I snuck into the bathroom (where I would spend a lot of time later on), drank it, and got off.

That thing that makes me different from normal people happened with that first beer. It felt really good. All those weird little childhood feelings went away, and I got off, man. I loved it immediately. I stumbled around the house in a euphoric buzz, and when that wore off, I puked my guts out.

But because I have this disease—I didn't know it at the time—I went back and got another one immediately. It kicked off a 20-year run.

The first illegal drug I ever did was LSD. I was nine. Man, I had a great time. I spent all day tripping, hanging out with my grandpa. He was a kind, old, stoned-out alcoholic guy. He sat there all buzzed out, and I lay on the floor, watching it melt. I didn't know it then, but the hits I took were supposed to be split between four people. There were no consequences. I didn't get caught. I loved it. I started smoking pot right after that. I'd heard drugs were bad, but my experience was that nothing bad happened. For me, it felt good, and I wanted to keep doing it for a long time.

I smoked pot pretty much every day for 20 years. I started taking pills and discovered that I liked things that made me go down. When my grandmother died of lung cancer, I went into the bathroom and stole her liquid morphine. It was really great. I totally do not relate to the concept of "drug of choice." I'd never even heard that term before I walked into a treatment center and they asked me what mine was. I'm like, "What the hell's that?" I was a mixer. I liked to put four, five, or seven different things into my body to see what would happen.

For me, there was tons of pot and acid and all kinds of pills because everybody has a bathroom. I became the medicine cabinet bandit and had perfected the "cough-n-flush." I preferred those prescriptions that read "Do not take with alcohol" or "May cause drowsiness." I did that for a long time, which culminated with me taking poison that I thought was some kind of psychedelic and then running around the house naked, writing on the walls. My folks had to literally hold me down on the floor and sit on my back, I was so out of my mind. It was a scary thing. I figured the problem was the acid, so I eliminated it from my list of things I could do safely.

High school was all about being high. My coping skills in high school were eye drops, cologne, and gum; get rid of the bloodshot eyes, take the reek off, and chew some gum, man. That's what I needed to get by. I would sell a little bit of this or that, making friends because I always had a bag of pot.

We moved every couple years, so I was always going to a new school. But I could spot my people a mile away. Big boots, torn jeans, bandanas tied around the leg, leather jacket, smoking. There's my people. "You get high?" "Yeah." Best of friends immediately. We had something in common. I related to people by getting loaded.

I did my first line of cocaine in the bathroom at high school. I was so amped up playing basketball, I was practically passing the ball and running to catch it myself. It was really great. But for me, cocaine was expensive and hard to get, so it became an every once in a while kind of thing.

Somehow, I got into college. College was great. I ran around in the redwoods and got loaded, went to keg parties, snorted speed. Crank, now there's a nasty drug, right? I'd snort a line, tears running down my face, feeling like I'd just snorted battery acid. Then it would hit me, and I'd say, "This is great!" Four days later, when everybody is a cop, you know, it wasn't so much fun.

The progressive nature of this disease was really starting to come out for me. I didn't know that's what it was; I thought it was about "tolerance." I used to take great pride in my ability to out-party people. I'm the guy who could walk into a convenience store at 1:55 a.m. and deal with the lights. I did all that stuff I had to do to feel normal, but looking back, I can really see how those first two beers when I was nine were not what I needed to get the desired effect when I was 20.

Addiction is sneaky and subtle. It crept into my life and started taking hold of all these things that I liked to do, like create art, play sports, cook food, go dancing. It stole all of those things away, but so subtly, I actually thought I was making the decisions to not do them anymore.

When my life really started falling apart, I figured the problem was the town I was living in, so I started moving around. But I would always end up with myself, doing what I needed to do, and it would fall apart *again*, so I'd move *again.*

I found heroin through another friend. In my forever clever mind, I thought I was just going to try it once. A month later, I'm still trying it. Within a year, I wanted to stop with all of my might and absolutely could not. That failure reinforced what a piece of crap I was, along with all that guilt and shame that was beginning to weigh heavy on me. I was getting into things that caused me a lot of guilt, and I was spending all my money just trying not to be sick.

So my forever clever mind made another career choice. I decided to start camping. It saved money; I didn't have to pay rent. It was a great plan. My life went downhill really fast because suddenly I had cash in my wallet that didn't have to go for bills or rent. I migrated to the middle of a blackberry bush. I forgot skills like eating. I didn't brush my teeth or my hair or get a haircut. I certainly didn't bathe. My idea of doing laundry was hosing myself off fully dressed in someone else's backyard. I lost weight fast. I kept thinking I was putting on a good-looking outer shell even though I was dying inside.

I ended up living in that bush for quite a few years. Every year, it seemed like I'd drop a notch and worse things would happen; I used to say that my life was just in a slump. I'd go home for the holidays to recuperate. Eat, sleep, and bathe. I'd start feeling a little better, then go back out and repeat what I now understand to be a desperate experiment.

During those years, I was even able to stop using on many, many occasions. But I could not stay stopped. I would get through five days with not sleeping, diarrhea, vomiting. It would prove to me that I could stop anytime; therefore, I could shoot a little heroin "socially" on a Friday night. That would start it all over again. At the time, I had no idea what I was up against. Once I start, I don't stop when I want to. It was brutal.

I had also become increasingly lonely. I couldn't be around anyone. I was unbelievably, painfully alone, and it crushed me. Every morning I'd wake up and say, "I don't want to do this again today. I don't want to do this again today." But I felt so bad, and the mental obsession was ruling my life, so I would go and do it again. Then it was, "Oh, you loser! You did it again!" I desperately tried to stop through all sorts of methods: therapy, moving, reading inspirational books ... everything.

Finally, my family held an intervention. In my forever clever mind, I came up with "my" program. I went to a couple of meetings to get everybody off my back. I was still smoking pot and was miserable, not doing any of the work. I would sit in the back of the meeting and leave as soon as it was over. I'd go home and drink a pint.

I went through a second, professional intervention and agreed to go into a treatment center. I tried to be a star pupil, convinced that knowing what was wrong with me was going to help me. It didn't. What did happen was that there were these H&I meetings coming in to the treatment center, and they planted the seed of hope in me. I didn't realize it at the time. At the time, I'd hear, "I haven't drank or used in 10 years." And I'd go, "Yeah, right. It can't be done. Look at you. You've got a watch. You've eaten today. And you're far too happy!"

But way in the back of my brain, I started to think that maybe, just maybe, one of these people wasn't lying. That's when I started to understand.

I had learned a little about the progressive nature of this disease. I knew how much I was doing before I started treatment and how much I was still doing, seemingly against my will. I was breaking into houses, ripping off my friends. I was doing all these terrible things that I hated doing, and from the outside, it looked like I didn't care. But I'm an addict with a huge heart, and I cared, and I wanted to do the right thing. I just couldn't do it. My addiction was ruling my life, crushing me.

This went on for about six or seven months. I was living in the woods, hadn't bathed in about a month, and was eating a burrito a week. I had to wake up with two needles in each arm just to not be sick. It had long since stopped being a party.

One day, there in the woods, I felt something shift in my heart. I felt something move, and the feeling behind it was that the honeymoon was over. I knew I could not do this anymore.

What came out of my mouth was something that I'd never said before, not even in desperation. Oh, I'd done a lot of "God, if you get me out of this, I promise I'll never ... " praying to the porcelain God and that kind of thing, but this was different. This came from my soul. I said, "God, please help me!"

I remembered those people from H&I talking about how they asked for help from something greater than themselves. Now I prayed for help.

Then the cops showed up. Not exactly what I had in mind. I saw this cop a ways off, walking on the railroad tracks. I believe today that God just walked me right up to this guy. Of course, I snapped out of it when he threw me in the back of the police car in handcuffs, but it was too late.

Jail was a good place for me to think. My first 30 days, I didn't sleep or eat. I lay on the floor like a pile of laundry. That was about all I could do, other than crawl to the bathroom. When I was offered the opportunity to get bailed out, I don't know why, but I refused.

When I got out of jail, I was ready to do this thing. I decided that if I didn't like what happened at the end of the Twelve-Step process, I'd go out and drink and use again. I went into a treatment center, and once again, they told me to get a sponsor, work the Steps, and go to meetings. This time I did that. And my life changed unbelievably.

I started with a meeting that became my home group. In that meeting and for the first time in my life, I said, "I have no idea how to stay clean and sober. I have no idea how to live without putting something in my body. How do I do this? Can you guys help me?" There were about six dudes, and they made recovery look so cool to me. These guys said, "Do what we do, and you will get what we have." I really wanted what they had.

Then I got busy with the Steps. I learned that the first thing is for me to know in my innermost being that I have this disease and to acknowledge that I'm never going to be cured, meaning that I can never safely drink or use again for the rest of my life. How do I do that? I started by hanging with "us" every day. I learned in the First Step that as long as I could fully concede that I am never cured, then I might be able to admit that I'm powerless. That's what I did. I learned that lack of power was my problem, and as a result, my life was unmanageable. I had been sleeping under a bush for years; it was not a big stretch for me to come to that realization.

I struggled with the Second Step. I did not think of myself as insane. There was a time when I would punch myself in the face in order to go to doctors to get painkillers. I'd punch myself in front of the mirror until I had a nice, swollen head. "Normal" people probably don't do that crap, but it made sense to me. Once, while taking care of two young children, I had drugs sent to me by overnight shipping. I didn't have a rig, so with my forever clever mind, I manufactured one by sharpening a basketball inflation valve. I'm trying to jam this thing into my arm with no veins left, and I'm responsible for two little kids. That was the kind of willingness I had to go get loaded. Yet I did not consider it as insanity because no one got hurt. So I struggled with the idea that I needed sanity to be restored to my life.

Finally, it was pointed out to me that insanity is not the stupid crap I did out there when I was getting loaded; it's the idea that I could continue to get loaded successfully. It's my forever clever mind that convinces me that despite the thousand times that previously ended horribly, it would be different this time. Insanity is doing the same thing over and over again and expecting different results. Or for me, knowing what the results would be and doing it anyway. I learned through this Step process that being sane means that when I occasionally get that thought now, I don't believe it.

I love the Third Step. I love the Third Step Prayer. I'm a big believer in it. In the first two Steps, I got to look back in my history and learn some things about myself. Step Three is where I get to start moving forward. It is where I get to learn how to get out of my own way. I had learned that I am my own problem. I'm selfish, and this selfishness was going to kill me. I also learned that God would help me get rid of it. My experience is that the longer I work to do my best to turn my will and my life, my thoughts and actions over to the care of a Higher Power, the more I care about other people, and the less selfish I am. My selfishness still returns an awful lot. I frequently wake up thinking about myself, and if you ever see me doing something nice for somebody, it's because I've been thinking about myself. That's what I was taught to do—go out and help somebody, get out of my own way.

The Fourth Step scared me until I'd done it and experienced the relief it offered. If you're new in recovery and you haven't done it, it's actually pretty simple. In four columns, I listed the people I was ticked off at, what they did, how that affected me, and in the fourth column, identified my part. I got to that column, and I was like, "Huhhhh?" I had never, ever considered that I had a part. I was a victim when I got here, and I'm not a victim today. I have a role in every single situation I put myself into.

So I made my list of resentments. I did a list of fears, and I took a good hard look at my sexual inventory and discovered why I pushed people away and why I get involved. I learned an awful lot by taking stock of myself.

Then I shared it all with my sponsor in a Fifth Step. And he laughed. Ticked me off, man. I'm reading him all this stuff, pouring my heart out to him, and he's just cracking up, laughing until tears were running down his face. I'm like, "A—hole!" He says, "No, bro, I'm relating!" Then he shared his experience back to me, and I went, "Wow, you're really sick, man!" Immediately, I felt a little bit better. I had that sense of relief, like dropping a big, old backpack of weight. That was the first real unloading of all this guilt, shame, fear, and remorse that I'd been carrying around, and I didn't even know until I had put it all out in the light. I started to feel like there was some hope for me.

From the last column of my Fourth Step, I looked at what I wanted to keep and what I wanted to try and get rid of, identifying my defects of character. I learned the Seventh Step Prayer. I thought all I would have to do is say the prayer, and they'd all be gone—cool! I know better today; this is the stuff I get to work on for the rest of my life. But the edges have been rounded off, and I get to claim a little progress in some of those areas. Honestly, for me, there are even a few that, with God's help, have been removed entirely. God is pretty powerful. I believe that God can do anything.

In the Eighth Step, I made a list of people I owed amends and what I did. There was all the real obvious stuff, like, "I stole your TV and abused your trust," and then all the real subtle things, like trying to be nice to get my way. When I got really honest with myself, my list got fairly long.

So now with my list, I set out, absolutely willing to make amends to those people. My sponsor told me to start with some easy ones to get warmed up. But the next day my mom called and said, "Hey, we're coming into town." So I got the opportunity to make some of the more difficult amends first, individually to each of my parents.

There are still some people that I have to make amends to, and as long as I continue to have the willingness, God often puts them in my path. I've had old friends or girlfriends find my name in the phone book and just call me up. My experience is that my amends never work out the way I think they will; I talk, and then they talk, and then we have healing around a new relationship. I'm really grateful for that.

I love Steps Ten, Eleven, and Twelve. If I'm watching myself on a daily basis, cleaning up my side immediately and asking God for help, it is absolutely impossible for me not to change. If I'm seeking to improve my conscious contact with God, as I understand Him, through daily prayer and meditation, change is inevitable. I'm a big believer in prayer and meditation, and I wasn't before I got here. For me, meditation can be short, little moments or nice, long moments of quieting my mind. I love the word "improve" in Step Eleven.

I learned that if I work the first eleven Steps, I will have a spiritual awakening. As a result of working the Steps, I had one. It wasn't what I thought it would be. Not the skies parting, beams of golden light, angels singing. It's the stuff I get to do from the second I wake up in the morning. It's that I'm awake these days. It's the opportunity I have to try to do the next right thing, and how I'm a different human being because of it. It is an awakening that continues for me every day.

Service has been huge for me. I got a coffee pot commitment early on at my home group. It became an opportunity to get out of myself, to think about other people, and to build some self-esteem. It's a special thing to be able to give something back. I'll always be in debt because the more I do, the more I get.

I also work with others, and every time I take somebody through the Steps, I learn more about myself. I get a deeper understanding of how to apply these principles in all of my affairs, and I try to get a little bit better at doing it.

Being a product of H&I, I'm a big believer in it. I spend a lot of time going to treatment and detox centers. It puts things into perspective for me because I can relate to the guy sitting there in his foamy slippers, his eyes going different directions, shaking and sweating. And every once in a while, I meet somebody with two days, and then I'll see them years later, and they're still continuously sober, they've worked the Steps, they're a sponsor, and they have a sponsor. It's an amazing process.

I honestly believe that because we can relate to each other, one addict to another, we have the ability to reach out and grab hold of each other and to save each other's lives. Because we can gain each other's trust when nobody else can. Because we can show each other how to do this thing.

I think it's like elephants. I'm an old stoner, and I like those nature programs. So I think it's like elephants. They line up behind the oldest matriarch, holding onto the tail of the elephant right in front of them. And they follow each other, using the collective wisdom and the old-age experience. I honestly believe that's how this whole thing works, one person following the next. It's a very special, wonderful, beautiful thing. It's truly a blessing in my life. I feel honored and privileged to be a part of it.

26

MOMENT OF CLARITY

An experience of conscious contact removed his obsession to use.

As of this writing, it has been over 20 years since I last used drugs or alcohol. If I'd thought I might live to write about it, I would have taken more pains to make my drug addiction more entertaining. If it's disheartening to read, well, it was worse to live it.

I was born in the mid-1950s to an affluent couple who were perfectly suited to raise me. My father was a career alcoholic in the middle of making his third fortune in the oil industry. He had already drank up the other two fortunes. He drank up the third one as well, come to think of it. My mother was possessed with her own neuroses and fears that covered most of her day-to-day existence. Materially, I wanted for nothing. I was born with the proverbial silver spoon in my mouth, which later on moved upwards towards the nostril.

Problems started to surface at an early age for me, somewhere around five. I found friendships with other people bewildering. The hand I was dealt in this life was intelligence, family wealth, and cowardice. After enough drugs were consumed, intelligence was reduced considerably. Family wealth was dissipated nicely by my father. That left me with cowardice, which is the personality characteristic that dominated me for the first 27 years of my life. My experience with cowardice is that it is what results from exposure to constant fear. It also goes away after about six lines of good cocaine. For a while, anyway.

I became a drug addict in about 15 minutes one rainy Tuesday. I had been sampling legal and illegal drugs for a number of years before I became an addict. I drank to get drunk. I smoked hash to oblivion. I had eaten LSD. None of those things controlled me. I could take it or leave it at the time. However, I had never tried cocaine. One of the people I grew up with dealt cocaine occasionally. I mentioned to him that next time he got some, I'd like to buy some.

A couple of months went by, and then I got a phone call. At that time, cocaine was pretty pricey, and I asked how much it cost. When I was told, my thought was that it was an awful lot of money for a little dab of white powder.

I also remember having a little quiet thought way deep in my gut: "Do you *really* want to try this?" I brushed the thought aside with, "Of course I do. There isn't anything I can't handle."

So, I went home with my little purchase in hand and instructions for use. I tried some, and nothing happened. I tried some more. Still nothing. So, I threw the remainder in the top drawer of my toolbox in the garage and promptly forgot about it for three months. Sort of like putting a hand grenade in your pocket with the pin halfway pulled out.

Three months goes by, and I find myself working on a race bike in my garage on a rainy Tuesday. I was racing off-road during those years, and it was an obsession with me. It was about to be replaced with another obsession. I ran across the little package of white powder and wondered if it was still any good. I thought maybe I hadn't used enough of it before, so I snorted half of it.

Twenty minutes later, I was sitting there, looking at the mirror, thinking, "Where have *you* been all my life?"

I only snorted one line of cocaine after that. It was almost six years long. It almost killed me a number of times. Towards the end, I wished it would.

The effect of my first suicide attempt with cocaine was dramatic, to say the least. As the rush started, I had a very bad feeling. I suddenly began sweating profusely, my knees began trembling, and I couldn't stop twitching. In my right eye, a light began flashing, in time with my heart rate. After a moment, I began to see images in the flashes of light, like they were caught by a strobe light. Images from my life. All of it.

After a short while, the flashes became breathtakingly fast, and it felt like a blow to my solar plexus. I was above my body, watching it convulse. There was no pain, only a deep sadness. I remember looking at my body twitching and thinking, "Poor bastard, he never had a chance."

The next thing I was aware of, I was lying on the floor, my jaws and eyes were black and blue, and I was incontinent. Such an overwhelming experience had a deep and profound effect upon me. I at once stopped using cocaine. For about 20 minutes. Then I resumed for over four years.

I finally reached the end. I was sleeping on a couch in my nephew's apartment. At six foot two, I weighed 164 pounds. It was the night of my last suicide attempt. I headed to the beach. I had a plan. I was going to snort the last of my cocaine on the end of the pier, and when the rush hit, I was going head first into the sand 60 feet below. I'd turn my head just before I hit, and that should do it. It was 1 a.m., and the pier was deserted.

God has a sense of humor and will always touch you in a way you can understand. As I got up on the rail and was looking down, I had this thought: "You are such a screw up, you'll just break your neck and be a vegetable for the next 40 years. You couldn't even kill a crippled animal properly."

Being the coward that I was, I climbed off the rail and wandered back to the couch I was living on. Sitting there at 3 a.m., burnout time, I saw this 10-second public address spot on the TV: a voice saying, "Had enough?" and the image of a hand crushing up a short length of drinking straw. And a phone number. Nothing else.

I wrote the number down on a matchbook cover and put it in my wallet, but I was too scared to call. It took a month to get up the courage to dial the number. And another few days to actually leave a message.

An hour after leaving the message, I got a call back. It was the first time in my life I had ever talked to someone who had been where I was and lived to tell about it. He gave me the time and address of a C.A. meeting for that night. On the way home from my third trip to my dealer's that day, I stopped in at the C.A. meeting. I had an eight ball half gone in my pocket and hadn't showered or slept in four days. I listened to what people said. Then someone lit a candle on a cake, and a guy who said he was a surgeon stood up and celebrated a period of one year without any drugs. From where I stood, that looked like the peak of a distant mountain.

I went home that night, finished the eight ball, and made a decision. I'd gone cold turkey before and knew that I'd have a seizure if I stopped cold. So, I drew a line in the sand, so to speak, at a friend's housewarming party that was coming up, and I began cutting in half the amount I did each day. The party came, and I announced to the people standing around, as I put a very large line on the mirror, "This is the last line you will ever see me snort."

They all laughed at me. With good reason. I could have had any odds I wanted in a bet on that statement. They had all seen me use and knew it was impossible for me to quit.

But I haven't had a line since that day. It's been 20 years. So far, so good.

I can assure you I had stopped hundreds of times before. Why did this one stick? In short, I had an experience of conscious contact with God at 28 days sober. At that time, the obsession to use cocaine was removed. It has never returned.

Cocaine Anonymous was having their first spiritual retreat, and I was the newest newcomer in attendance. Saturday night during a meeting, I felt very strange and went outside. I got into my car and drove out into the middle of the desert. I started crying, couldn't stop, and ended up on my knees by the side of the road, in the middle of the desert, in the middle of the night, and I prayed like I'd never prayed before. The only word I could say was "Please." I didn't even know what to ask for. I was so alone, and so scared.

The next moment, there was a warm feeling in the pit of my stomach, and it spread outward from there. I saw in a split second my whole life before me, and it was ugly. Then, all of a sudden, the ugliness was gone, and a very gentle, quiet voice inside of me said, "You are free."

And I was.

I drove back to the retreat and walked into the meeting room. There were people still sitting and talking, and I walked in with tears streaming down my face. I said, "I know a lot of stuff, but I don't know anything important." It was the beginning of learning for me. I was 28 years old, and the scope of my ignorance about everything spiritual and emotional was limitless.

A week or so later, with some guidance, some paper, and a pencil, I reached the Ninth Step of the Twelve-Step process. It took three and a half hours. At the end of that time, I had, in my own handwriting, a list of things I had to do. If I did them, I would remain sober. If I didn't, I'd use. It was as simple as that. I got busy. Fences needed mending, so to speak, and there wasn't much time. I had between that instant and my next line to get through Step Nine. I did much of it in a day and a half. It took a few years to make the financial restitution.

A couple months later, I was at work, talking to God as I worked, and I didn't agree with how God was handling a number of things in my life. My prayer went something like this: "God, I need to know exactly what is going on with these things that are bothering me, and I need an answer, and I need it pretty damn quick!"

I went back to work, and maybe 10 minutes later, my pager beeps. It shows the number to call, and I don't recognize the number. So I drop a dime in the pay phone and dial the number. It's a church that I've never heard of before, and it's their dial-a-prayer line. The recorded message answers every question that I'd been asking a few minutes before.

I am stunned. After listening to the message for a few times, I call the number of the church office given at the end of the message and explain what happened, and the lady on the end of the line says, "Yeah, we get stuff like that happening all the time. Kinda neat, huh?"

So I mention I am a member of a Twelve-Step group, and the lady says, "Oh, we have meetings here." And this little voice in my gut says, "They don't have any C.A. meetings." It took a month for me to get one started there.

Today in my life, this whole Twelve-Step process distills down to three things for me. First, I continue to perform a written inventory, and when I am wrong, I correct it as soon as possible. Second, I pray and I meditate. In all honesty, meditation is something I do more than prayer. It's more important to me to learn how to listen; I already know how to talk. Finally, having had a spiritual awakening as the result of these Steps (prayer, meditation, and an honest written inventory), I try to practice this way of living in all my affairs and to pass on this way of living to anyone who might benefit from it.

The Twelve-Step process removed the fear I had lived under all my life, and a side benefit was that my drug addiction simply disappeared. It was absolutely effortless.

Today I bear no resemblance to that person who set out to kill himself with cocaine. I'd have to say that I've given my life to become the person that I am today, and it's been worth it.

Something that I shared at that first Cocaine Anonymous retreat bears repeating: for everything that I might be, and for everything that I might not, I'd like to thank all of you for my life.

LITERATURE

1	COCAINE ANONYMOUS SELF-TEST	197
2	TIPS FOR STAYING CLEAN AND SOBER	201
3	THE FIRST 30 DAYS	203
4	A HIGHER POWER	207
5	THE HOME GROUP	209
6	CHOOSING YOUR SPONSOR	213
7	BEING OF SERVICE	217
8	CRACK	221

1

COCAINE ANONYMOUS SELF-TEST

It is the collective experience of the members of Cocaine Anonymous that addiction is a problem not limited to cocaine or any other mind-altering substance. With this in mind, we suggest you answer the following questions:

1. Have you ever used more cocaine, alcohol or other drugs than you planned?
2. Has the use of cocaine, alcohol or other drugs ever interfered with your job?
3. Is your use of cocaine, alcohol or other drugs causing problems within your relationships?
4. Do you ever feel depressed, guilty, or remorseful after using cocaine, alcohol or other drugs?
5. Do you use whatever cocaine, alcohol or other drugs you have, almost continually, until the supply is exhausted?
6. Have you ever experienced physical problems due to your use of cocaine, alcohol or other drugs?
7. Do you ever regret using cocaine, alcohol or other drugs for the first time?
8. Do you ever obsess about getting cocaine, alcohol or other drugs when you do not have any?
9. Are you experiencing financial difficulties due to your use of cocaine, alcohol or other drugs?

10. Do you experience an anticipation high when you are about to use cocaine, alcohol or other drugs?

11. Do you have difficulty sleeping without alcohol or other drugs?

12. Are you absorbed with the thought of using cocaine, alcohol or other drugs even while interacting with a friend or loved one?

13. Have you begun to use cocaine, alcohol or other drugs while you're alone?

14. While using or drinking, do you ever have feelings that people are talking about you or watching you?

15. Do you have to use more cocaine, alcohol or other drugs to get the same effects you once experienced?

16. Have you tried to cut down on your use of cocaine, alcohol or other drugs only to find that you could not?

17. Have you tried to stop using cocaine, alcohol or other drugs only to find that you could not stay stopped?

18. Have any of your friends or family suggested that you may have a problem with cocaine, alcohol or other drugs?

19. Have you ever lied to or misled people about how much cocaine, alcohol or other drugs you use?

20. Have you ever lied to or misled people about how often you get high or drunk?

21. Do you use cocaine, alcohol or other drugs in your car, at work, in the bathroom, or in other public places?

22. Are you afraid that if you stop using cocaine, alcohol or other drugs, your work will suffer or you will not be able to function?

23. Do you spend time around people or go places you would normally stay away from if not for the availability of cocaine, alcohol or other drugs?

24. Have you ever stolen money, cocaine, alcohol, or other drugs from friends or family?

25. Has using and/or drinking cost you more than money?

If you have answered "yes" to any of these questions, you may have a problem. There is an answer: Come to meetings of Cocaine Anonymous. While the name "Cocaine Anonymous" may sound drug-specific, we wish to assure you that our program is not. Many of our members did a lot of cocaine; others used only a little, and some never even tried coke. Whether we focused on a specific mind-altering substance or used whatever we could get our hands on, we had one thing in common: eventually we all reached a point where we could not stop. Over time, virtually every single one of us has realized that our real problem is not cocaine or any specific drug; it is the disease of addiction.

According to C.A.'s Third Tradition, the only requirement for membership is a desire to stop using cocaine and all other mind-altering substances. It doesn't matter to us if you drank or what type of drugs you used; if you have a desire to stop, you are welcome in Cocaine Anonymous!

2

TIPS FOR STAYING CLEAN AND SOBER

Here are some tips to help you.

- Admit that you lack the power to stay clean on your own.
- Make sobriety your #1 priority.
- Throw away all your drugs and drug paraphernalia.
- Don't deal drugs.
- Go to meetings daily.
- Get phone numbers and use them.
- If your dealer calls, hang up and call someone on your phone list.
- If no one is home and you're in trouble, call the C.A. helpline.
- Stay away from people, places and things with which you associate drug use.
- Choose a home group; let people get to know you.
- Get a sponsor and call your sponsor every day.
- Work the Twelve Steps of Cocaine Anonymous with your sponsor.
- Read the books and literature.

- Be of service; get a commitment at a meeting.

- Be honest, open-minded and willing (H.O.W.).

- Don't get too hungry, angry, lonely or tired (H.A.L.T.).

- Keep it simple. We stay clean and sober one day at a time.

- Pray. Ask questions. Seek answers.

- No matter what happens, keep coming back!

- Be patient. Recovery takes time.

- Remember, we care.

3

THE FIRST 30 DAYS

WELCOME to Cocaine Anonymous. We are all here for the same reason—our inability to stop using cocaine. The first step towards solving any problem is understanding the problem.

THE PROBLEM The problem, as we see it, consists of an obsession of the mind and a compulsion of the body. The obsession is a continued and irresistible thought of cocaine and the next high. Once we have given in to this thought, our bodies take over. Our compulsion consists of an absolute inability to stop using once we begin. Thus, our recovery begins with complete abstinence from cocaine and all other mind-altering substances. This allows us to begin living in the solution.

THE SOLUTION We wish to assure you that there is a solution and that recovery is possible. It begins with abstinence and continues with practicing the Twelve Steps of recovery one day at a time.

Take it easy. Addiction is not a moral issue. Addiction is a disease—a disease that kills. Here are some suggestions to help you stay clean and sober for your first 30 days:

Abstinence – Do not use any mind-altering substances! Experience has shown us that the use of any mind-altering substance will ultimately lead us back to addiction in another form or to our drug of choice, cocaine.

A Meeting a Day – Attend at least one meeting a day–or more. Meetings are where we go to share our experience, strength, and hope with each other.

Get a Sponsor – It is a good idea to get a sponsor during your early days, when C.A. seems unfamiliar. A sponsor is simply a sober addict who can give you more time and attention than is available at meetings.

Use the Telephone – Get phone numbers from C.A. members and use them. A vital part of our recovery process is reaching out to others. If no one is available, call Cocaine Anonymous.

One Day at a Time – We stay clean and sober one day at a time, and, when necessary, one hour or even one minute at a time; not one week, or one month, or one year, just one day at a time.

As we get clean and sober, our feelings begin to surface. Cocaine helped us escape from ourselves; it altered our reality. It helped us cover up, avoid, and deaden our feelings. Getting clean and sober can be painful, but with help, we find our lives get better one day at a time.

When we attended our first C.A. meeting, we knew deep down inside that cocaine had become a problem in our lives. Seeing this was just the beginning. This is where the program of Cocaine Anonymous comes into play. We begin by surrendering and working the Twelve Steps of recovery.

STEP ONE: *We admitted we were powerless over cocaine and all other mind-altering substances—that our lives had become unmanageable.*

Most of us disliked the idea of being powerless over anything. We thought that cocaine made us invincible and powerful, when in actuality, it wiped us out financially, emotionally, physically, and spiritually. We were out of control and had reached the depths of despair. The extent to which our lives had become unmanageable, of course, was different for each of us. The fact remained that our lives had become unmanageable. Not until we got honest with ourselves and surrendered, did we begin to know peace.

STEP TWO: *Came to believe that a Power greater than ourselves could restore us to sanity.*

Step Two involves open-mindedness. Having admitted we were powerless over cocaine and all other mind-altering substances, we became open-minded enough to believe that a Power greater than ourselves could remove our obsession to use and restore us to sanity. The obsession to use will be removed. This Power may be, but does not have to be God. Many of us use the Fellowship of C.A. as our Higher Power. After all, what we had failed to do alone, we are succeeding in doing together.

STEP THREE: *Made a decision to turn our will and our lives over to the care of God* as we understood Him.

Cocaine Anonymous is a spiritual program, not a religious one. We claim spiritual progress rather than spiritual perfection. Some of us arrived with a God, while others used the group until they found a Higher Power of their own understanding. A key phrase in this Step is "*as we understood Him.*" In Cocaine Anonymous, each individual can choose a God of his or her own understanding.

As we worked the Twelve Steps of recovery, we began to see some of the Promises coming true in our lives:

> *If we are painstaking about this phase of our development, we will be amazed before we are halfway through. We are going to know a new freedom and a new happiness. We will not regret the past nor wish to shut the door on it. We will comprehend the word serenity and we will know peace. No matter how far down the scale we have gone, we will see how our experience can benefit others. That feeling of uselessness and self-pity will disappear. We will lose interest in selfish things and gain interest in our fellows. Self-seeking will slip away. Our whole attitude and outlook upon life will change. Fear of people and of economic insecurity will leave us. We will intuitively know how to handle situations which used to baffle us. We will suddenly realize that God is doing for us what we could not do for ourselves.*[7]

[7]This excerpt from Alcoholics Anonymous, pages 83-84, is reprinted with permission of Alcoholics Anonymous World Services, Inc. ("AAWS"). Permission to use this excerpt does not mean that AAWS has reviewed or approved the contents of this publication, or that AAWS necessarily agrees with the views expressed therein. A.A. is a program of recovery from alcoholism only—use of this material in connection with programs and activities which are patterned after A.A., but which address other problems or concerns, or in any other non-A.A. context, does not imply otherwise.

4

A HIGHER POWER

As a newcomer, you may have thought or said, "What's this talk about God? I came here to stop using cocaine, not to join a new religion." Don't feel alone. Many of us were put off with the talk about God when we first came to meetings.

It is easy enough to confuse the word spirituality with religion. As it relates to God, Cocaine Anonymous is a spiritual program, not a religious one. In C.A., we believe each individual can choose a Higher Power of his or her own. In short, a God of his or her own understanding.

If you are like many of us, you came to C.A. without a conscious belief in a Higher Power. Or, perhaps you chose to avoid a Higher Power because you were taught about a punishing God. It doesn't matter. All that is necessary to start is that you are open-minded to the idea that *some* Power greater than yourself may be able to restore you to sanity.

The first step in solving any problem is recognizing it. The same holds true in solving a problem with cocaine.

The second step in solving a problem is believing that there might be a solution. The fact that you've come to a C.A. meeting shows that you believe that there is a Power of some kind, greater than yourself, that can help you get your life back in order. You have proven, just by showing up, that you believe that there must be some information, somewhere, you can use to get rid of your obsessions with cocaine, drugs, and/or alcohol. You have already started!

The third step in solving a problem, after having found evidence of a solution, is putting faith in that solution and trying it. The solution for us meant admitting that our management of the problem wasn't working. Cocaine Anonymous introduced us to a Power greater than ourselves that *could* manage our problem. That doesn't necessarily mean we have to turn our will and our lives over to the care of the God that we heard of in the past. It can mean trusting in a Power of our own understanding. This is the beginning of our Higher Power, God as we understand Him.

Some of us adopt, or come back to, a traditional God. Others see our Higher Power as some kind of force. Some define it as the force of the group, while others don't define it at all.

At first, it is sufficient for God, as you understand Him, to be the power that the group obviously has to help get rid of the obsession to use.

No one comes into Cocaine Anonymous to find God. We come to these rooms to get rid of a terrifying drug habit. Look around in a meeting. You are surrounded by people who came as a last resort. We came into these rooms emotionally, financially, and spiritually bankrupt. We have experienced all sorts of tragedies as a result of cocaine, drugs, and/or alcohol. We have lived many of the same horrors you have, yet today we are happy. We are free from the misery, terror, and pain of drug addiction.

As long as you are willing, your belief will grow. You will learn through your own experience and the experiences of others how a Higher Power can help you with your cocaine problem.

Maybe some of us were worse off than you; maybe some of us didn't hit as low a bottom as you. Still, the fact remains, that those of us who are recovering have come to believe that the power of the group or of a Higher Power of our own understanding can restore us to sanity.

After you are around the program for a few weeks and months, you will begin to see changes in your thinking. You will begin to feel better. You will see changes in the other newcomers that came in with you. We call those changes miracles. If you are having trouble with the talk about God, remember:

- Be open-minded.
- C.A. is a spiritual program, not a religious one.
- All you have to do is to be willing to believe.
- Your Higher Power can be the group as a whole.
- You start with belief, your experience will come.

Don't leave before the miracle happens!

5

THE HOME GROUP

BECOMING PART OF

It is the common experience for many of us to feel like we didn't fit in anywhere. Drugs gave us that instantaneous feeling of belonging. When we get sober, that drug-induced feeling of belonging disappears. Finding a group of sober people we can relate to is a new start for us. We go to meetings as often as possible, preferably every day.

Before long, we find we are most comfortable at one particular meeting. Because we feel "at home" there, we join the home group and commit to attending regularly. Other home group members get to know who we are, and we get to know them. We never have to be alone again. On a bad day, we find there is usually someone there who understands and who can help us get through it sober.

THE HOME GROUP As newcomers, we hear the suggestion to get a "home group," but we aren't sure why. Many of us have been in isolation for the last months or years of our using. We feel apart from society and need to connect with people who understand. We find those people at meetings of Cocaine Anonymous.

TEMPORARY SPONSORSHIP Since our home group gets to know us quite well, they can sometimes act as our sponsor at the beginning of our recovery until we get one of our own. They give us suggestions and listen to our troubles. They explain what the Steps are for and may even get us started on the work. They give us hope to continue on our journey.

A POWER GREATER THAN OURSELVES Sometimes it is difficult to develop a concept of a Power greater than ourselves. Our drugs had been such a power, but what could be greater than that?

As we begin to work a program of recovery, we learn that we are defenseless against our addiction. We need a Power greater than ourselves, greater than our addiction. There may be no better place to start than with a group of sober addicts. Our own concept of a Higher Power will come in time as we work the Twelve Steps. Until then, it is good to have the power of the group with us.

TWELVE-STEP WORK / SERVICE We often wonder how we can carry the message to the addict who still suffers before we get through working all of the Steps. The answer is service. Wasn't it important to us to have someone at the door to welcome us? Was there coffee made? Did someone take the time to greet us? Were there chairs set up? Who read the readings at the beginning of the meeting? Was there someone to empty the ashtrays? We can find a way to help no matter how long we have been sober. We are told that getting out of ourselves is one of the best things for us to do, and serving our home group is a wonderful way to start.

RESPONSIBILITY In our active addiction, we were often irresponsible and unaccountable. We often placed blame on others and none on ourselves. Taking on responsibility at our home group is a good step forward. Although you probably won't become treasurer at your first business meeting, you might become the coffee person, showing up early to make sure the coffee is ready for the early birds and staying late to clean up the pots and cups. There are a variety of positions that need to be filled at most groups: Chairperson, Secretary, Group Service Representative (GSR), Greeter, Coffee Maker, Chips and Literature Representative, Floor Sweeper and others. All are very important. There is always something you can do, no matter how long you have been sober. Being of service at your home group is a great way to practice being a responsible member of society.

The benefits of becoming involved in a home group are more than you can probably imagine. It can be an important part of the process that ultimately keeps us clean and sober. One of our original members writes, "It occurred to me that when many of us walk through the doors of Cocaine Anonymous for the first time, we do so without hope, without faith, but with an ounce of *courage*. We listen to the stories and experiences of others and develop *hope*. As a result of coming back, and coming back, and coming back and working the Twelve Steps, we acquire an abundance of *faith*." (*Hope, Faith & Courage Volume II, page 6.*)

We encourage you to keep going to meetings until you find yourself a home group–and no matter what, keep coming back.

6

CHOOSING YOUR SPONSOR

WHY SPONSORSHIP? You've likely heard lots of talk at Cocaine Anonymous meetings about working the Twelve Steps of recovery, finding a Power greater than ourselves, and getting a sponsor. If you're like most newcomers, however, you're probably not sure what all these terms mean.

This is why it's a good idea to get a sponsor. A sponsor can devote individual attention to answering your questions regarding the C.A. program of recovery. It can also help you feel more comfortable to be with someone who knows his or her way around. A sponsor can introduce you to other C.A. members, help you get involved in service and encourage you to participate in Fellowship events, all of which are vital to a successful program of recovery.

We can benefit immensely from one-on-one support as we begin learning how to live in recovery. Many of us would not have been able to stay clean and sober were it not for the special relationship with our sponsor. Sharing difficulties with a sponsor makes the struggle less lonely and the day-to-day living a lot easier.

WHAT IS A SPONSOR? A sponsor is a recovering addict who shares one-on-one how to maintain sobriety by working the Twelve Steps of C.A. A sponsor's primary tools are his or her own experience, strength and hope. The Steps can seem like a foreign language at first, but a sponsor can help us understand this new way of living and explain how each Step brings us closer to a Higher Power that can remove our obsession to use.

Sponsors are not professional counselors and are not certified to offer legal, psychiatric or medical advice. Nor should we become dependent on our sponsors to get us jobs, clothing or food. However, sponsors may have experience with how to obtain professional help or other resources.

A DISCUSSION OF SPONSORSHIP There are no specific rules for sponsorship in C.A., but we do offer a few suggestions for your consideration.

Experience has shown that it's best to avoid the possibility of emotional and/or physical distractions that might take the newcomer's mind off the purpose of Cocaine Anonymous. For this reason, it may be wise to choose a sponsor of the same sex if we're heterosexual, and of the opposite sex if we're gay or lesbian.

Which sponsor is best for you? Only you can answer that question. You and your sponsor may have a lot in common or you may be totally different.

Sponsorship can involve a substantial amount of time and energy. To have a successful relationship, both parties should be willing to communicate on a regular basis.

It is also imperative that the sponsor provides a safe and supportive atmosphere. The sponsor should be careful not to share a sponsee's confidences with anyone else. This will help build a foundation of trust and encourage the sponsee to be honest. A sponsor needs to know what is truly going on in order to help the sponsee.

At times, we may feel uncomfortable with what our sponsor suggests. When this happens, it's important to remember that our sponsor has traveled the road before us and is sharing his or her experience to help us through difficult times.

It is your responsibility to call your sponsor, so do not hesitate to pick up the phone. It may be difficult at first to ask for help, but contacting your sponsor on a regular basis is one of the first ways you can take responsibility for your own recovery.

Remember, sponsors have lives outside of C.A. They have families, jobs and other responsibilities. There will be times when a sponsor is truly unavailable. When this happens, check the listings for the next local C.A. meeting, or perhaps join one of the online C.A. meetings. You could also read C.A. literature, contact the local C.A. helpline, or pull out your phone list. Keep an active list of recovering addicts' phone numbers with you at all times and above all CALL. Remember, our program is based on one addict helping another. The help is there, ready and willing to be shared, but you have to reach out and ask for it.

Working the Steps is not an overnight matter. It requires continuous action and a persistent look at the things that have blocked us from a Power greater than ourselves. Sobriety depends on maintaining fit spiritual condition, which we do by continuously working the Steps. This is why we suggest ongoing contact with a sponsor no matter how long you have been sober.

FINDING A SPONSOR Some of the ways we have found a sponsor are:

- Listening to and identifying with the feelings being shared at meetings;
- Noticing when someone has been where we have been and now has the kind of sober life we hope to have;
- Asking members of the Fellowship for their phone numbers, then calling between meetings;
- Sharing at meetings that we are looking for a sponsor;
- Asking other C.A. members to recommend a sponsor;
- Going to coffee after meetings with other C.A. members;
- Attending C.A. activities or events.

When choosing a sponsor, remember that this does not have to be a life-long relationship. Many of us have changed sponsors during the course of our sobriety. Others have had the same sponsor since early sobriety. The point is that YOU must take the initiative and reach out.

It is never too late to get a sponsor. Whether you are a newcomer hesitant about "bothering" someone, or a member who has been around for some time trying to go it alone, sponsorship is yours for the asking.

Most C.A. members owe their sobriety to the fact that someone else was willing to share a great gift with them. Getting a good sponsor, sharing honestly and listening to his or her experience can make the whole program open up as it never did before.

We in Cocaine Anonymous urge you: DO NOT DELAY. We want to share what we have learned with other addicts because experience has taught us that we keep what we have by giving it away. You will likely be helping your sponsor as much as your sponsor is helping you.

7

BEING OF SERVICE

In addition to finding a spiritual way of life, recovery is about changing negative aspects of our personalities into positive ones. We came into the program with big egos but little or no self-esteem. We thought we were better than other people yet, at the same time, felt "less than." We were people who took from others and abused friendships all of our lives. We had no concept of doing anything for anyone without the thought of some kind of reward. By the sheer grace of our Higher Powers, we have found several ways of unlearning such behavior in the program. One way is to be of service to the Fellowship of Cocaine Anonymous. We discovered that the best way to serve God was to serve our fellow humans, and we found humility in the process. Our self-centered behavior was gradually replaced with the "attitude of service." We learned that service is about gratitude and learning how to contribute to our lives and the lives of others.

Why Be of Service?

- To give back what was so freely given to us;
- To take on a commitment as a symbolic way of making amends;
- To meet other recovering addicts;
- To learn how to be part of a team;
- To learn humility by doing something selfless for someone else;
- To learn skills or teach others what we know;
- To learn responsibility.

Ways to Be of Service

Service Opportunities at the Meeting and Area Level:

Meeting Setup: Arrive early to set up chairs, make coffee, and greet newcomers.

Hotline: Did you find C.A. through a hotline? Answer the phones for your Area's hotline and be on the "front line" of helping others find C.A. and recovery.

Treasurer: Pass the 7th Tradition basket and keep track of funds for a meeting—it's a great way to learn responsibility.

GSR/DSR (Group/District Service Representative): Get involved in the business aspects of C.A. by representing one of your meetings or Districts at your District/Area business meeting.

Secretary: Ensure that a meeting will always be there for those who need it by choosing speakers, paying the rent, and keeping it running smoothly and consistently. You might even consider helping the Fellowship grow by starting a new meeting.

Committees at the Area and/or World Service Level:

Convention: Help plan big sober parties and carry the message of recovery at the same time.

Literature: If you have writing skills or ideas that could reach out in print to people who are still suffering, express those ideas on this World Service committee.

Finance: Put your accounting, business, or money management skills to good use in C.A.'s financial matters.

Public Information: Reach out through the media to those who have never heard of C.A.

Hospitals & Institutions: Help develop new ways to reach out to people who are unable to reach out for themselves.

Unity: Enhance communication and outreach among the diverse elements within our Fellowship.

Structure & Bylaws: Formulate bylaws, guidelines, and structures by which C.A. can operate.

Conference: Help organize the World Service Conference each year, where delegates from all over the world meet to conduct C.A. business.

Area & World Service Office Boards of Directors: Serve as a Chairperson, Vice-Chairperson, Secretary, Treasurer, or Director at Large. Conduct the day-to-day business operations of C.A. to ensure that it is there for newcomers the way it was there for you.

Ask your GSR who you can contact for more information about how to be of service.

Suggestions

- Share a commitment, such as a hotline slot, if your schedule doesn't allow you to have one of your own.
- Find a place where you can be of service and then give 100%.
- Volunteer at a meeting when help is asked for or better yet, before it is asked for.
- Encourage the people you sponsor to take on commitments and then help them to keep those commitments.
- Ask your sponsor what type of service commitment you could take on that would best serve the Fellowship.
- Adopt the attitude of service without reward.

Remember, time spent working on a commitment is time not spent getting loaded.

8

CRACK

"At first it was fun. Then it reached the point where every time I used, I had chest pains and my heartbeat would go crazy; and yet I couldn't stop."

"There I lay in the hospital, almost dead from an overdose. My heart felt like it was about to jump out of my chest and yet all I could think about was getting another hit."

"I couldn't stop until my whole paycheck was gone. I promised myself that next week it would be different—'I'll only do one'—but one turned into two, two turned into three, and before I knew it, I was promising myself again: 'Next week it will be different ... '"

"I had it all—a good job, a loving wife and family, everything I ever wanted and WHAM! It was all gone in a matter of weeks."

"I said that I would never be caught peeping out windows or crawling around on the floor. A few days later I was peeping and geeking. I thought someone was out to get me. The paranoia almost drove me insane."

"I knew it was killing the baby growing inside me, but I couldn't stop. I couldn't stop and then it was too late and I still couldn't stop."

"At first it was gotta quit; then it was gotta quit, can't quit; can't quit, gonna die."

Can you relate to these feelings? Have you been through many of the same situations, made the same promises to your family, to your friends, and most of all, to yourself?

So have we. We have truly wanted to keep these promises. We did everything in our power, but we still always seemed to come up short.

Who are we? We are former crack users. We are members of Cocaine Anonymous.

Today, many of us realize that crack cocaine played a major role in our failures and in our broken promises. We know that cocaine took away our drive to do anything except more cocaine. We were driven by cocaine and nothing else seemed to matter. Even if it made us feel miserable, we had to have it.

If crack cocaine made us feel miserable, why did so many of us continue to use? Ask a hundred cocaine addicts that same question and you will probably get a hundred different answers, but no matter how many reasons exist, one fact is certain: crack cocaine is a highly addictive drug. Once used, it becomes the root of most of our problems.

For many of us, it was only a matter of weeks of using before our whole world came crashing down upon us; for some it came sooner, for some it came later. Some of us used other drugs or alcohol for years without ever experiencing the loss that we experienced with crack cocaine.

SO HOW DO WE STOP USING CRACK?

Cocaine Anonymous has a few simple suggestions on how you should start:

ABSTINENCE Don't use no matter what. We suggest abstinence from all mind-altering substances.

ONE DAY AT A TIME Remember that you don't have to stay clean and sober for the rest of your life. We do this one day at a time.

MEETINGS Attend C.A. meetings daily. Cocaine Anonymous meetings are where you meet other recovering addicts who have similar problems. We share our experience, strength, and hope with each other to find common solutions through working the Twelve Steps of Cocaine Anonymous.

TELEPHONE When you want to use, call the Cocaine Anonymous hotline in your area. Get phone numbers from people in the meetings and call them day or night.

Remember that you are not alone. Keep in touch with other recovering cocaine addicts. We are here to help you.

WE'RE HERE AND WE'RE FREE™

APPENDICES

A	SUGGESTED PARTICPATION MEETING FORMAT	227
B	TWELVE STEPS OF COCAINE ANONYMOUS	241
C	TWELVE TRADITIONS OF COCAINE ANONYMOUS	243

A

SUGGESTED PARTICIPATION MEETING FORMAT

Welcome to the (________) meeting of Cocaine Anonymous. My name is (________) and I am an addict. Are there any other addicts present? Welcome! Not to embarrass you, but so that we could get to know you better, will those of you in your first 30 days of sobriety please let us know who you are? Would you please stand and state your name and your disease? If you're visiting from out of town or new to the Area, please introduce yourself.

Cocaine Anonymous is a Fellowship of men and women who share their experience, strength and hope with each other that they may solve their common problem and help others recover from their addiction. The only requirement for membership is a desire to stop using cocaine and all other mind-altering substances. There are no dues or fees for membership; we are fully self-supporting through our own contributions. We are not allied with any sect, denomination, politics, organization, or institution. We do not wish to engage in any controversy and we neither endorse nor oppose any causes. Our primary purpose is to stay free from cocaine and all other mind-altering substances, and to help others achieve the same freedom.*

We use the Twelve Steps of recovery because it has already been proven that the Twelve-Step recovery program works.

It is a custom in Cocaine Anonymous to read *We Can Recover*, taken from the C.A. "Storybook." I've asked (________) to read for us.

The Twelve Traditions are to the group what the Twelve Steps are to the individual. I've asked (________) to read for us.

*Adapted with permission of the A.A. Grapevine, Inc.

(OPTIONAL: It is also a custom to read *Who is a Cocaine Addict? Who is a C.A. Member?*, or *Alcohol*. I have asked (________) to read for us.)

(OPTIONAL: LEADER QUALIFIES FOR 5-10 MINUTES) This is a 1½-hour participation meeting. We encourage newcomers to ask any questions they may have regarding the program and recovery. Please do not share if you have had any drugs or alcohol in the last 24 hours. There is no cross-talk at this meeting, and all questions should be directed at the speaker. Please limit your sharing to 3-5 minutes. Who would like to start?

(FIVE MINUTES BEFORE COFFEE BREAK) We are fully self-supporting through our own contributions. At this time we will observe the 7th Tradition. Newcomers need not feel obligated to contribute. Please remain quietly seated while the baskets are being passed.

(AFTER BASKETS ARE COLLECTED) We will now have a 5-minute coffee break.

(AFTER COFFEE BREAK)

(OPTIONAL) We give chips at this meeting for 30, 60 and 90 days, 6 and 9 months, 1 year, 18 months, and 2 or more years of continuous sobriety—free from all mind-altering substances. Please keep your sharing brief so that we may have time for participation afterward. Is there anyone here in their first 30 days of sobriety who wishes to take a newcomer chip? 30 days? 60 days? 90 days? 6 months? 9 months? 1 year? 18 months? 2 or more years?

We give a cake for every 365 days of continuous sobriety. We have (________) birthdays.

Now we will continue with participation.

(TEN MINUTES BEFORE THE MEETING ENDS) Our time is up. If you have any questions that went unanswered, or if you feel the need to share, please introduce yourself to someone after the meeting and exchange phone numbers. We are all here to help. Are there any secretary's announcements?

(AFTER SECRETARY'S ANNOUNCEMENTS) I would like to close by having (________) read *The Promises, A Vision for You,* or *Reaching Out.*

After a moment of silent meditation for the addict who still suffers, would (________) lead us in the prayer of his/her choice?

WE CAN RECOVER

Welcome to Cocaine Anonymous. We are all here for the same reason—our inability to stop using cocaine and all other mind-altering substances. The first step towards solving any problem is admitting that there *is* a problem.

The problem, as we see it, consists of an obsession of the mind and an allergy of the body. The obsession is a continued and irresistible thought of cocaine and the next high. The allergy creates an absolute inability to stop using once we begin.

We wish to assure you that there *is* a solution and that recovery *is* possible. It begins with abstinence and continues with practicing the Twelve Steps of recovery, one day at a time. Our program, the Twelve Steps of Cocaine Anonymous, is the means by which we move from the problem of drug addiction to the solution of recovery.

1. We admitted we were powerless over cocaine and all other mind-altering substances—that our lives had become unmanageable.

2. Came to believe that a Power greater than ourselves could restore us to sanity.

3. Made a decision to turn our will and our lives over to the care of God *as we understood Him*.

4. Made a searching and fearless moral inventory of ourselves.

5. Admitted to God, to ourselves, and to another human being the exact nature of our wrongs.

6. Were entirely ready to have God remove all these defects of character.

7. Humbly asked Him to remove our shortcomings.

8. Made a list of all persons we had harmed, and became willing to make amends to them all.

9. Made direct amends to such people wherever possible, except when to do so would injure them or others.

10. Continued to take personal inventory and when we were wrong promptly admitted it.

11. Sought through prayer and meditation to improve our conscious contact with God *as we understood Him*, praying only for knowledge of His will for us and the power to carry that out.

12. Having had a spiritual awakening as the result of these Steps, we tried to carry this message to addicts, and to practice these principles in all our affairs.[8]

Cocaine Anonymous is a spiritual program, not a religious one. In C.A. we believe each individual can choose a Higher Power of his or her own. In short, a God of his or her own understanding.

No one comes into Cocaine Anonymous to find God. We came into these rooms to get rid of a terrifying drug habit. Look around this room. You are surrounded by people who came as a last resort. We came into these rooms emotionally, financially and spiritually bankrupt. We have experienced all sorts of tragedies as a result of cocaine, drugs and/or alcohol. We have lived many of the same horrors you have, yet today we are free from the misery, terror and pain of addiction.

Maybe some of us were worse off than you; maybe some of us didn't hit as low a bottom as you. Still the fact remains that those of us who are recovering have come to believe that a Higher Power of our own understanding can restore us to sanity.

There *is* a solution; we *can* recover from addiction. One day at a time, it is possible to live a life filled with hope, faith and courage.

[8]The Twelve Steps are reprinted with permission of Alcoholics Anonymous World Services, Inc. Permission to reprint and adapt the Twelve Steps does not mean that A.A. is affiliated with this program. A.A. is a program of recovery from alcoholism. Use of the Steps in connection with programs and activities which are patterned after A.A. but which address other problems does not imply otherwise.

THE TWELVE STEPS OF ALCOHOLICS ANONYMOUS:1. We admitted we were powerless over alcohol—that our lives had become unmanageable. 2. Came to believe that a Power greater than ourselves could restore us to sanity. 3. Made a decision to turn our will and our lives over to the care of God *as we understood Him*. 4. Made a searching and fearless moral inventory of ourselves. 5. Admitted to God, to ourselves, and to another human being the exact nature of our wrongs. 6. Were entirely ready to have God remove all these defects of character. 7. Humbly asked Him to remove our shortcomings. 8. Made a list of all persons we had harmed, and became willing to make amends to them all. 9. Made direct amends to such people wherever possible, except when to do so would injure them or others. 10. Continued to take personal inventory and when we were wrong promptly admitted it. 11. Sought through prayer and meditation to improve our conscious contact with God *as we understood Him*, praying only for knowledge of His will for us and the power to carry that out. 12. Having had a spiritual awakening as the result of these Steps, we tried to carry this message to alcoholics, and to practice these principles in all our affairs.

THE TWELVE TRADITIONS

1. Our common welfare should come first; personal recovery depends upon C.A. unity.

2. For our group purpose there is but one ultimate authority—a loving God as He may express Himself in our group conscience. Our leaders are but trusted servants; they do not govern.

3. The only requirement for C.A. membership is a desire to stop using cocaine and all other mind-altering substances.

4. Each group should be autonomous except in matters affecting other groups or C.A. as a whole

5. Each group has but one primary purpose—to carry its message to the addict who still suffers.

6. A C.A. group ought never endorse, finance, or lend the C.A. name to any related facility or outside enterprise, lest problems of money, property and prestige divert us from our primary purpose.

7. Every C.A. group ought to be fully self-supporting, declining outside contributions.

8. Cocaine Anonymous should remain forever nonprofessional, but our service centers may employ special workers.

9. C.A., as such, ought never be organized; but we may create service boards or committees directly responsible to those they serve.

10. Cocaine Anonymous has no opinion on outside issues; hence the C.A. name ought never be drawn into public controversy.

11. Our public relations policy is based on attraction rather than promotion; we need always maintain personal anonymity at the level of press, radio, television and films.

12. Anonymity is the spiritual foundation of all our Traditions, ever reminding us to place principles before personalities.

 THE TWELVE TRADITIONS OF ALCOHOLICS ANONYMOUS: 1. Our common welfare should come first; personal recovery depends upon A.A. unity. 2. For our group purpose there is but one ultimate authority—a loving God as He may express Himself in our group conscience. Our leaders are but trusted servants; they do not govern. 3. The only requirement for A.A. membership is a desire to stop drinking. 4. Each group should be autonomous except in matters affecting other groups or A.A. as a whole. 5. Each group has but one primary purpose—to carry its message to the alcoholic who still suffers. 6. An A.A. group ought never endorse, finance, or lend the A.A. name to any related facility or outside enterprise, lest problems of money, property and prestige divert us from our primary purpose. 7. Every A.A. group ought to be fully self-supporting, declining outside contributions. 8. Alcoholics Anonymous should remain forever nonprofessional, but our service centers may employ special workers. 9. A.A., as such, ought never be organized; but we may create service boards or committees directly responsible to those they serve. 10. Alcoholics Anonymous has no opinion on outside issues; hence the A.A. name ought never be drawn into public controversy. 11. Our public relations policy is based on attraction rather than promotion; we need always maintain personal anonymity at the level of press, radio and films. 12. Anonymity is the spiritual foundation of all our Traditions, ever reminding us to place principles before personalities.

WHO IS A COCAINE ADDICT?

Some of us can answer without hesitation, "I am!" Others aren't so sure. Cocaine Anonymous believes that no one can decide for another whether he or she is addicted. One thing is sure, though: every single one of us has *denied* being an addict. For months, for years, we who now freely admit that we are cocaine addicts thought that we could control cocaine when in fact it was controlling us.

"I only use on weekends," or
"It hardly ever interferes with work," or
"I can quit, it's only psychologically addicting, right?" or
"I only snort, I don't base or shoot," or
"It's this relationship that's messing me up."

Many of us are still perplexed to realize how long we went on, never getting the same high we got at the beginning, yet still insisting, and believing—so distorted was our reality—that we were getting from cocaine what actually always eluded us.

We went to any lengths to get away from being just ourselves. The lines got fatter; the grams went faster; the week's stash was all used up today. We found ourselves scraping envelopes and baggies with razor blades, scratching the last flakes from the corners of brown bottles, snorting or smoking any white speck from the floor when we ran out. We, who prided ourselves on our fine-tuned state of mind! Nothing mattered more to us than the straw, the pipe, the needle. Even if it made us feel miserable, we had to have it.

Some of us mixed cocaine with alcohol or other drugs, and found temporary relief in the change, but in the end, it only compounded our problems. We tried quitting by ourselves, finally, and managed to do so for periods of time. After a month, we imagined we were in control. We thought our system was cleaned out and we could get the old high again, using half as much. This time, we'd be careful not to go overboard. But we only found ourselves back where we were before, and worse.

We never left the house without using first. We didn't make love without using. We didn't talk on the phone without coke. We couldn't fall asleep; sometimes it seemed we couldn't even breathe without cocaine.

We tried changing jobs, apartments, cities, lovers—believing that our lives were being screwed up by circumstances, places, people. Perhaps we saw a cocaine friend die of respiratory arrest, and *still* we went on using! But eventually we had to face facts. We had to admit that cocaine was a serious problem in our lives, that we *were* addicts.

Reprinted from the C.A. pamphlet *To the Newcomer*.

WHO IS A C.A. MEMBER?

While the name "Cocaine Anonymous" may sound drug-specific, we wish to assure you that our program is not. Many of our members did a lot of cocaine; others used only a little, and some never even tried coke. We have members who drank only on occasion, those who casually referred to themselves as drunks, and others who were full-blown alcoholics. Lots of us used a wide variety of mind-altering substances. Whether we focused on a specific substance or used whatever we could get our hands on, we had one thing in common: eventually we all reached a point where we could not stop.

According to C.A.'s Third Tradition, the only requirement for membership is a desire to stop using cocaine and all other mind-altering substances. ***Whatever you may have been using, if it led you to this meeting, you're probably in the right place***. Over time, virtually every single one of us has realized that our real problem is not cocaine or any specific drug; it is the disease of addiction.

It can be tempting to focus on our differences rather than our similarities, but this can blind us to potential sources of support in our recovery. As we hear other members' stories, the most important question to ask ourselves is not, "Would I have partied with these people?" but rather, "Do these people have a solution that can help me stay sober?" We encourage you to stick around and listen with an open mind.

With its all-inclusive Third Tradition and First Step, Cocaine Anonymous welcomes anyone with a drug or alcohol problem and offers a solution. C.A.'s Twelve Steps are not drug-specific, and Cocaine Anonymous is not a drug-specific Fellowship. It doesn't matter to us if you drank or what type of drugs you used; if you have a desire to stop, you are welcome here!

ALCOHOL

Alcohol is a mind-altering substance in liquid form. Many people don't realize it is no different from cocaine or other drugs in its ability to lead to addiction. One drink is never enough, just as one hit, fix, pill or snort is never enough. We are masters at combining and substituting one drug for another to get high. Many of us never felt that alcohol was part of our problem.

THE PROMISES

If we are painstaking about this phase of our development, we will be amazed before we are half way through. We are going to know a new freedom and a new happiness. We will not regret the past nor wish to shut the door on it. We will comprehend the word serenity and we will know peace. No matter how far down the scale we have gone, we will see how our experience can benefit others. That feeling of uselessness and self-pity will disappear. We will lose interest in selfish things and gain interest in our fellows. Self-seeking will slip away. Our whole attitude and outlook upon life will change. Fear of people and of economic insecurity will leave us. We will intuitively know how to handle situations which used to baffle us. We will suddenly realize that God is doing for us what we could not do for ourselves.

Are these extravagant promises? We think not. They are being fulfilled among us—sometimes quickly, sometimes slowly. They will always materialize if we work for them.

A VISION FOR YOU

Our book is meant to be suggestive only. We realize we know only a little. God will constantly disclose more to you and to us. Ask Him in your morning meditation what you can do each day for the man who is still sick. The answers will come, if your own house is in order. But obviously you cannot transmit something you haven't got. See to it that your relationship with Him is right, and great events will come to pass for you and countless others. This is the Great Fact for us.

Abandon yourself to God as you understand God. Admit your faults to Him and to your fellows. Clear away the wreckage of your past. Give freely of what you find and join us. We shall be with you in the Fellowship of the Spirit, and you will surely meet some of us as you trudge the Road of Happy Destiny.

May God bless you and keep you—until then.

REACHING OUT

I made it into this program because someone else worked their Twelfth Step on me. Someone passed it on to me. Someone was out there after they got clean and sober, caring about others. I need to never, ever forget that. Had they simply gone on with their lives and forgotten about people like me who were still out there using and suffering, I wouldn't be here today. My gratitude begins with that fact. It is with that gratitude in mind that I reach out to others, especially the newcomers. I need to have them in my life. That is where my spirituality begins.

For me, spirituality comes from caring about others. I have found that the more I focus on improving the quality of the lives of others, the less I am into myself and my will. I feel a freedom and peace from within. The gifts I am beginning to receive in my life are greater than I could have ever imagined.

Something else I have done is that I have forgiven myself. I have forgiven myself for being an addict. I have forgiven myself for all the damage I did to my life, to my physical health, and to my career and finances. But most of all, I have forgiven myself for all of the horrible, negative and unloving things I have felt about myself. It was not until I offered and accepted my own forgiveness, that I was truly able to grow in my sobriety.

B

TWELVE STEPS OF COCAINE ANONYMOUS

1. We admitted we were powerless over cocaine and all other mind-altering substances—that our lives had become unmanageable.
2. Came to believe that a Power greater than ourselves could restore us to sanity.
3. Made a decision to turn our will and our lives over to the care of God *as we understood Him*.
4. Made a searching and fearless moral inventory of ourselves.
5. Admitted to God, to ourselves, and to another human being the exact nature of our wrongs.
6. Were entirely ready to have God remove all these defects of character.
7. Humbly asked Him to remove our shortcomings.
8. Made a list of all persons we had harmed, and became willing to make amends to them all.
9. Made direct amends to such people wherever possible, except when to do so would injure them or others.
10. Continued to take personal inventory and when we were wrong promptly admitted it.
11. Sought through prayer and meditation to improve our conscious contact with God *as we understood Him*, praying only for knowledge of His will for us and the power to carry that out.
12. Having had a spiritual awakening as the result of these Steps, we tried to carry this message to addicts, and to practice these principles in all our affairs.

C

TWELVE TRADITIONS OF COCAINE ANONYMOUS

1. Our common welfare should come first; personal recovery depends upon C.A. unity.
2. For our group purpose there is but one ultimate authority—a loving God as He may express Himself in our group conscience. Our leaders are but trusted servants; they do not govern.
3. The only requirement for C.A. membership is a desire to stop using cocaine and all other mind-altering substances.
4. Each group should be autonomous except in matters affecting other groups or C.A. as a whole.
5. Each group has but one primary purpose—to carry its message to the addict who still suffers.
6. A C.A. group ought never endorse, finance, or lend the C.A. name to any related facility or outside enterprise, lest problems of money, property and prestige divert us from our primary purpose.
7. Every C.A. group ought to be fully self-supporting, declining outside contributions.
8. Cocaine Anonymous should remain forever nonprofessional, but our service centers may employ special workers.
9. C.A., as such, ought never be organized; but we may create service boards or committees directly responsible to those they serve.
10. Cocaine Anonymous has no opinion on outside issues; hence the C.A. name ought never be drawn into public controversy.
11. Our public relations policy is based on attraction rather than promotion; we need always maintain personal anonymity at the level of press, radio, television and films.
12. Anonymity is the spiritual foundation of all our Traditions, ever reminding us to place principles before personalities.

 THE TWELVE TRADITIONS OF ALCOHOLICS ANONYMOUS: 1. Our common welfare should come first; personal recovery depends upon A.A. unity. 2. For our group purpose there is but one ultimate authority—a loving God as He may express Himself in our group conscience. Our leaders are but trusted servants; they do not govern. 3. The only requirement for A.A. membership is a desire to stop drinking. 4. Each group should be autonomous except in matters affecting other groups or A.A. as a whole. 5. Each group has but one primary purpose—to carry its message to the alcoholic who still suffers. 6. An A.A. group ought never endorse, finance, or lend the A.A. name to any related facility or outside enterprise, lest problems of money, property and prestige divert us from our primary purpose. 7. Every A.A. group ought to be fully self-supporting, declining outside contributions. 8. Alcoholics Anonymous should remain forever nonprofessional, but our service centers may employ special workers. 9. A.A., as such, ought never be organized; but we may create service boards or committees directly responsible to those they serve. 10. Alcoholics Anonymous has no opinion on outside issues; hence the A.A. name ought never be drawn into public controversy. 11. Our public relations policy is based on attraction rather than promotion; we need always maintain personal anonymity at the level of press, radio and films. 12. Anonymity is the spiritual foundation of all our Traditions, ever reminding us to place principles before personalities.